# Free Yourself From Hot Flushes and Night Sweats

## The Essential Guide to a Happy and Healthy Menopause

### By Silvana Siskov

# Thank you for purchasing
## *Free Yourself From Hot Flushes and Night Sweats: The Essential Guide to a Happy and Healthy Menopause*

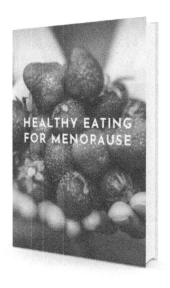

Please visit <u>bit.ly/menopause-healthy-recipes-1</u>
and download
*Healthy Eating for Menopause – Recipe Book.*

You will find plenty of delicious recipes there
to help you achieve a confident body.

# Table of Contents

# Introduction

The menopause is a challenging stage in a woman's life.

Some women have an easier time than others, but most women struggle at one point or another. There is a range of common symptoms during the menopause, and without a doubt, hot flushes and night sweats are up there as the most commonly experienced ones.

It is easy to assume that the menopause is a natural process; therefore, you just have to "put up" with the symptoms and wait for the storm to pass. But these days women do not have to let the menopause to control them. There are many approaches to take that can reduce the effects that menopausal symptoms have on your life. Very often, making small changes to your lifestyle can be enough to take the edge off the severity of troublesome symptoms you experience and allow you to go about your life more easily.

The aim of this book is to help you understand the reasons behind the most common menopausal symptoms, and then talk you through the ways you can reduce their effect on your life. You will discover that the majority of the symptoms can be reduced by focusing on a healthier approach to life. This would include cutting down on smoking and reducing alcohol intake, consuming a healthy diet packed with clean, fresh produce and a variety of vitamins and minerals, doing your best to get enough sleep, and including more exercise in your lifestyle. Many symptom treatment methods are often interlinked, so focusing on a healthier life overall will give you a head start in coping with several troublesome menopausal symptoms.

Overhauling your lifestyle may not be necessary. Perhaps you already exercise regularly, but you need to focus on your diet a little more. Maybe you do not drink or smoke, but you need to learn to find the time to exercise. People live their lives in many different ways, though there are healthy changes every woman can make to her lifestyle which can have far-reaching effects on her health and well-being, as well as her management of her menopausal symptoms.

Finding the time to exercise does not need to take a massive chunk out of your day. It can be just 20 to 30 minutes in the morning or during the evening. Eating a healthier diet and learning to cook, instead of ordering takeaways, is not too hard to achieve when you change your mindset and take on a new approach to dieting, and in this book I will show you how to do that. It can even save you money and be an enjoyable experience.

Focusing on health and well-being is your number one route towards a healthy and happy menopause.

Throughout this book, you will discover the role of hormones and how they affect you. I will give you information on why menopausal symptoms occur and what to do about them. Knowledge is power, and understanding what is going on in your body during this time of your life will provide you with the confidence to reduce the effects of its symptoms and alleviate any worries you may have.

In the first chapter of this book, I will give you some general information about the menopause to help you understand what is going on inside your body. Then, I will talk about the main symptoms and why they happen. You will see a recurring theme throughout this chapter and learn the leading cause of every symptom you experience.

There are over 30 menopausal symptoms, but it is worth remembering that not every woman is going to have the full list of symptoms that the menopause can bring.

By understanding why you experience particular symptoms and learning how to reduce them, you are giving yourself the best possible chance of achieving a healthier and happier experience. You may also be able to pass on your newly acquired knowledge to friends and family members who are also going through the menopause.

The remainder of the chapters will be dedicated to investigating specific common symptoms, exploring why the menopause happens and providing practical advice on how to reduce its effects naturally, wherever possible. I will also explain about hormone replacement therapy (HRT), a hot topic among women approaching and going through the menopause. HRT is a contentious subject and the one that you need to fully understand if you want to take advantage of its benefits — if you choose to do so.

It is a good idea to read through every symptom guide, because even if you are not dealing with it right now, it does not mean you will not in the future, and besides, focusing on optimal health is never a bad thing.

The menopause is very challenging, and at times you will be tired, you will be stressed out, and you will feel down. However, this book will give you the information you need to overcome those effects and feel far better as a result. There is no need to struggle alone and there is no need to assume that you just have to deal with it yourself. There is a lot of help out there. You will simply need to look for it, and in some cases, just ask for it.

The advice contained within this book will give you back the power to deal with this challenge you are faced with. You can then shape your response to the menopause in any way you see fit, owning your menopause, rather than allowing the menopause to own you.

# Chapter 1

# The Menopause Explained

Welcome to the first chapter!

The fact that you have read the book to this point means that you are interested in learning more about the menopause, how to deal with the symptoms, and how to reduce their impact on your life.

Before we delve into the symptoms and how to handle them better, I must give you some background information. You probably already know a little about what the menopause is, why it happens, and the types of things that can occur during this time. However, it is unlikely that you know it all. That is where this chapter is going to help you out.

In the following chapter, I will dive deep into the main menopausal symptoms and explain why you may experience them by exploring what is going on inside your body to cause them. But for now, let's look at what is going on inside your body generally at this time. Remember, knowledge is power!

# Hormones and Their Key Role

If you are wondering why you are feeling hot, cold, sweaty, tired, anxious, agitated, or why you cannot sleep, it is mainly because of your hormones. Hormones are the thing that women have been battling with since day one.

When we are young, usually in our teens, our body prepares us for the ability to reproduce, and at this time, we experience our first major hormonal shift. As young women, we develop breasts, our hips widen, and we start our menstrual cycle. Each girl experiences this period of growing up and becoming a woman in her own way and in her own time.

Later, when we reach a certain age, our genetic matter is no longer at its prime to reproduce, so our bodies decide that it is time for us to stop procreating. Due to hormonal shifts that become more pronounced over time, our bodies are no longer able to carry a new life through pregnancy and safe delivery.

During this time, our hormones experience a significant change that might impact not only on our physical health, but also on our mental and emotional health. Therefore, it is vital to incorporate nutrition, physical activity, and even potentially a talking therapy to offer us well-being and emotional support through this period.

The power of hormones is enormous! Everything about how the body operates is connected to the delicate balance of hormone production. If you give your body the nutrition, activity, sleep, and peace of mind that it needs, it is designed to provide you with health in return. You get back what you put in!

The fluctuation of hormones during the menopausal phase might disrupt your body, causing a difference in your weight and affecting sleep patterns and your sex drive, among other factors. This is natural, normal and safe, and it does not have to be unbearable. However, if your hormones are confused because of regular yo-yo dieting and environmental disruptors, the changes you experience will be unnatural and will likely feel uncomfortable and perhaps cause some lasting damage too. Significant weight gain, particularly around your mid-section, unpredictable hot flushes, mood swings, and other symptoms of menopause, can be tempered when your body finds its natural balance again.

As you become older, your body creates increasingly lower amounts of female hormones, and as a result, the menopause begins. Here are the three main hormones which gradually diminish with age, causing you to experience menopausal symptoms:

- Oestrogen

- Progesterone

- Testosterone

Testosterone is a male hormone, but women also produce it and need it in small amounts.

As I have already mentioned, hormones are extremely powerful, which is why they have such a significant effect on some women and the way they feel. Hormones control a considerable number of functions within the body and they can lead to the development of certain conditions.

For instance, you may be at risk of developing osteoporosis in later life because of less oestrogen. Lack of oestrogen might make your bones weak and less flexible. You may also feel far less like having sex with your partner because you have less testosterone in your body, affecting the way you think, feel, and your general libido. Changes in hormones can also cause you to gain weight in specific areas during the menopause, usually around the midriff and abdomen.

The reduction of these critical hormones is the reason you are going through this change in life and why you might be feeling like you are going through hell.

Menopause may be a fact of life for all women, but it does not have to be a tragic health condition that is unavoidable. Normal and average do not necessarily correspond to natural or healthy, and there is a way to navigate through the menopause without having your entire life disrupted. Thankfully, we are going to talk about that in much more detail as we move through the book.

## When Does the Menopause Happen?

If you search for the definition of the menopause, you will find something along the lines of "ceasing of menstruation". That means that your periods come to an end, and your body no longer releases an egg every month. You no longer bleed because you are not pregnant, and you no longer can become pregnant naturally. The good news is that you no longer have to deal with period cramps and other rather annoying symptoms that you have experienced for the last 30 or so years.

The menopause is a slow and steady process and often begins from around the age of 45 to 50 on average. However, you should not use those ages as a hard and fast guideline, because every woman is different. Some women start going through it much later, and others experience it much earlier.

There is a theory that women generally follow the pattern from their mothers. If your mother went through the menopause at the age of 45, for example, you would do the same. However, there is no concrete evidence to back this up. It is sometimes useful to look at your family history to predict the behavior of your genes, but in this instance, it might not be helpful. You can have a family of two sisters, one of them may follow the mother's pattern, whilst the other may be far younger or far older when her menopause begins. This has certainly been the case with my family.

The period before your menopause properly begins is called the perimenopause. This roughly translates to "around the menopause", so the time leading up to the actual point when you stop menstruating properly. During the perimenopausal stage, you might have a whole myriad of different symptoms. You will probably still have a monthly period, although sporadically, heavily or lighter than usual, and experience a range of other things that often fall into the perimenopausal "normal" range. It is not unusual for a woman's periods to become lighter, heavier, more irregular, more frequent, vary from spotting to heavy bleeding, and then back again. It is almost impossible to predict a pattern for your periods.

The perimenopause can last up to 10 years or so before the menopause is established. This is when you stop releasing eggs and stop menstruating. At this point, you are no longer fertile and can no longer become pregnant naturally. Symptoms can continue for another 10 years, although in most cases they will not be as severe. Remember, these are general patterns and must be heeded with caution, as every woman is different.

You should consider yourself as being through the menopause, i.e. postmenopausal, after you have not had a period at all for one year and are over the age of 50. If you are under the age of 40, you will need to be clear of periods for two years solidly, to be considered postmenopausal.

## What About Premature Menopause?

If you go through the menopause before the age of 40, you are classed as having a premature menopause. It is thought that around 5% of women go through the menopause early, therefore falling into this premature bracket.

Understandably, premature menopause can be extremely upsetting for a woman, especially if she still hopes to have a family or extend the family she already has. There is no reliable indicator of whether a woman is likely to go through the menopause early; again, it could be that if her mother did, she would be more likely to follow suit, but this has not been proven.

There are some risk factors for having premature menopause, including:

- Women who suffer from chromosomal problems, e.g. Turner syndrome

- Women who suffer from autoimmune conditions (in rare cases however)

- Genetic – Again, if a female member of your close family went through premature menopause, you may be more likely to do so, but not certainly

- Cancer treatments, such as chemotherapy or radiotherapy, may cause premature menopause for some women

- Women who have had surgery to remove one or both ovaries

Premature menopause is sometimes called premature ovarian failure. The symptoms are the same as those experienced by an "average aged" menopausal woman. If you do go through premature menopause, you will probably be advised to take HRT (hormone replacement therapy), and this is something I will discuss in more detail a little later.

## The Menopause is a Personal Deal

There is no denying that the menopause can be a challenging time for some women. On the other hand, some women sail through it and barely notice anything. It is a very personal deal and as a result, you should never compare your symptoms with a friend or a family member and then feel like there is something wrong with you if they do not match up.

Many women struggle with the fact that going through the menopause means that they are getting older. We cannot stop time, and getting older comes to us all, men included. So yes, the menopause is a sign of aging, but it is also a process that a woman's body needs to go through, and this does not make you any less attractive, or less feminine, or less powerful, or any less of a woman. If anything, it might even make you more of a woman, because you have taken on the ups and downs of the menopause and come out on top!

The menopause has the power to affect a woman's confidence in different ways; it can affect how you feel about yourself, your future, your appearance, and depending upon the age at which you go through the menopause, it might even mean that you have to come to terms with the fact that you are no longer able to carry a child of your own. The good news is that confidence can be built back up over time and a large part of handling the menopause and its symptoms is down to learning about the psychological and emotional effects.

Never be afraid of reaching out to those around you and talking about how you feel. If that is a little too close to home for you, find support in women your age, perhaps through social media or community support groups. You do not have to go through the menopause alone, and there is a lot of help and support out there if you reach out and ask.

This is your journey and one you should embrace as your own. In the rest of this book I will go into detail about some of the most common menopausal symptoms you might experience such as hot flushes, night sweats, lack of sex drive, headaches, etc., and give you plenty of advice on not only how to understand them, but also how to take them on and win!

## Key Points

- The menopause happens to every woman. This is the time when periods stop, due to the ovaries no longer releasing eggs.

- The start of the menopause is called the perimenopausal period and can begin at any time between 45 to 50 years old.

- Some women experience premature menopause, which means they begin the menopause before the age of 40.

- The menopause is established when a woman has not had a period for one full year if she is over 50.

- If you experience the menopause in your forties or earlier, you would need to be clear of periods for two years to be considered menopausal.

- The postmenopausal period (after you have reached the menopause) can still cause symptoms, and these may last up to 10 years in some cases.

- Menopausal symptoms are caused by dwindling hormone levels, namely oestrogen, progesterone and testosterone.

- The menopause can affect a woman's self-confidence, as well as causing troublesome or upsetting symptoms.

- The menopause is unique for each woman and can create different issues for each of us.

# Chapter 2

# An Overview of Common Menopausal Symptoms

Now you know what the menopause is and why it happens. It is time to move on to the very crux of this book — the symptoms you might experience, why you might experience them, and what you can do to reduce their impact upon your life.

There is a range of different symptoms which many women experience during this time. Sometimes the symptoms are more prevalent during the perimenopause, whilst other women notice far more symptoms during the actual menopause itself. Even after menopause has been established, e.g. in the postmenopausal period, it is entirely normal to have some of the symptoms for up to around 10 years afterwards. There is no hard and fast rule to adhere to here, and it is partly about going with the flow and understanding what is going on inside your body and allowing nature to do what it needs to do.

You might feel as though you have zero control and that you are at the mercy of your hormones. I understand that. But believe me, you have more say in this than you realise; you can reduce the severity of most symptoms by changing your lifestyle and by thinking about different treatment methods.

## Every Woman is Different

It is important to mention that every woman is different. Just because your friend, mother, sister, or anyone else experiences one particular symptom, that does not mean you are bound to. You might have a totally different set of symptoms from them. Your symptoms could be more severe or significantly less severe. You are a unique individual, and that means that your symptoms and your menopause might be slightly different or very different as a result.

Comparing your menopausal journey against another woman is not always useful because it can cause anxiety and worry if your experience is different, but the truth is that you are just going through your menopausal journey in your own unique way. Of course, if you are worried about something or if your symptoms become difficult to handle, you should definitely reach out to your doctor or another health professional to seek clarity and reassurance.

In the next chapter, we will talk about a few medical routes you could take, such as HRT, but for now, let's focus on the possible symptoms that may come your way, or in some cases, may not. We are going to look at why they are possible during this time and you will quickly see a pattern emerging; hormones are responsible for many ups and downs that you experience.

## The Importance of Understanding What is Happening to Your Body

Before we get onto the specifics, there is one other thing you need to know: You have to know what is going on inside your body to understand how to deal with it in a healthy way. When you do not know why something is happening, it is easy to worry over it. You might start panicking whenever you experience it, even though it could be a common menopausal symptom and not something that should trigger anxiety. Worrying can further compound the symptoms you are experiencing. It is far better to arm yourself with knowledge and understand your body better as a result of it.

You can empower yourself by learning about the common symptoms and understanding why they are happening. Only then can you take control of the menopause.

It is essential to understand that sudden changes in your body temperature, sleepless nights, mood swings, brain fogs, and terrible headaches, can be put down to your hormones. Though you might not be directly aware of them, hormones have great power and the ability to change the way you think, act, and feel.

You may have found that your emotions or mood have not been taken seriously in the past and you have probably heard phrases like "oh, she's just hormonal", or "it's her hormones again." I find it disrespectful to hear these things, and I know that many women struggle to accept these sorts of comments. Hormones have the power to affect our physical, emotional, and mental health, whilst causing a myriad of symptoms which are very hard to connect.

To create a significant difference in your health and well-being, it is crucial to focus on lifestyle changes to make things easier for you. I am not saying that all your symptoms will suddenly disappear, but improving your health will likely reduce the impact of menopausal symptoms on your life, and some of those symptoms will gradually fade and will not return. When you focus on healthy living and start looking after your body, you will notice many positive changes happening to you on a physical, emotional, and psychological level. This is something we are going to talk about in far more detail as we move through the book.

# Common Menopausal Symptoms and Why They Happen

Now, we are going to start getting to the real heart of the matter — menopausal symptoms and why they happen to us in the first place. As I have already mentioned, understanding why you are experiencing a specific symptom will allow you to feel calmer about it and then work out ways to control and minimise it, or possibly even remove it altogether.

Right now, I want to give you an informational overview of many menopausal symptoms that you might be experiencing, as it is important to get a broad view of what is happening to you at this time in your life. Then we are going to break your knowledge down into more distinct groups so you can get a better understanding of the range of symptoms that menopause can bring your way. In the coming chapters of this book, the focus will be on one specific symptom at a time and divided into different ways to control it.

I suggest that you do not skip any parts of the book and read all the chapters. All of the symptoms that I am going to discuss are common menopausal symptoms. Even if you are not experiencing some of the symptoms, you might find a useful piece of information and advice in this book which could help you live a healthier life in general.

Did you know there are over 30 menopausal symptoms that women can experience? So, what are the most common menopausal symptoms? Here is the list:

- Weight gain, specifically around the abdomen and midriff

- Hot flushes

- Night sweats

- Mood changes and irritation

- Fatigue

- Hair loss

- Anxiety

- Reduced libido

- Vaginal dryness

- Weak bones

- Brain fog

- Changes to the menstrual cycle, which then stop completely

- Problems sleeping

- Palpitations

- Headaches

- Focus and concentration problems

- Increased frequency of UTIs

- Thyroid issues

Before you panic, yes, that is a long list, but it does not mean you are going to experience all of those symptoms. Some women do, some do not, some have a few, some have half or more. Again, you are a unique individual, so we do not know what symptoms you may or may not have to deal with. It would not be unusual to start with one set of symptoms and then develop several more along the way; some might dwindle and disappear, only to come back a few months or a few years later. There is no pattern and no way of predicting which symptoms you may experience. You can only go with the flow and address what is in front of you.

I want to spend some time now informing you about the thyroid and its effects on your body because there is a strong connection between the menopause and thyroid disorder.

The thyroid is a small gland that sits at the front of your neck, just under what we call the "Adam's apple". The reason for thyroid issues to be quite common during this time of your life is that the thyroid comes under lots of pressure, due to the hormonal imbalance in your body.

You see, all the hormones work together and affect each other continuously. The thyroid is part of the endocrine system and it creates and releases two specific types of hormones, thyroxine and triiodothyronine. Both hormones are essential for ensuring the healthy functioning of the cells inside your body, and these hormones are also affected by other hormones. You already know that oestrogen, progesterone, and testosterone are reduced as the menopause approaches. As a result, this can sometimes cause problems with your thyroid and the treatment might be required to regulate and balance the hormones created and secreted by the thyroid.

Thyroid disorder is a complex condition that requires input from your doctor. The way to diagnose it is by taking your blood sample. Your doctor might ask you for the TSH test, T4 test, T3 test, and thyroid antibody test. These tests can show how well your thyroid is performing or how badly. Depending on the results, you might be prescribed a medication.

Many thyroid problems symptoms are very similar to the menopausal symptoms, and lots of women might be suffering from issues related to their thyroid disorder, but may think it is down to the menopause instead. Here are the most common symptoms of a thyroid disorder:

- Feeling tired a lot of the time

- Forgetfulness

- Putting on weight or losing it without trying

- Anxiety

- Feeling too hot or too cold

- Aches and pains in the joints and muscles

- Irregular periods

- Hair loss

- Dry and itchy skin

- Low mood

- Problems with concentration

Do you see the similarity between these symptoms and the symptoms of the menopause? That is why so many women fail to reach out to get treatment for their thyroid. They feel it is a part of their menopausal journey. My advice is, listen to your body and reach out if you suspect there may be a problem. You know your body better than anyone else and you should tune in and listen to what it is telling you. If your doctor does not take what you are saying seriously and you are concerned that something is not quite right, push the issue and ask for more tests. You are well within your rights to do so.

I would like to share my story with you now. I suffered from ill health for about five years from my late thirties to the early forties. I felt tired, had trouble sleeping, and I was losing my hair. Eventually, my periods started to become irregular. During this time, I visited a doctor regularly, until I was diagnosed with an underactive thyroid, a condition where the thyroid gland does not produce enough hormones.

I was prescribed medication for this condition, which I will probably take for the rest of my life, but this did not stop my troublesome symptoms from affecting me. During the perimenopausal phase my problems continued. Having an underactive thyroid and going through the perimenopause at the same time, I was never quite sure which of my symptoms were caused by the thyroid issue and which ones were triggered by the perimenopause, as they share many common symptoms.

Research shows that low levels of oestrogen caused by the menopause can significantly affect the thyroid hormones, but there are also suggestions that thyroid disorder can cause the menopause to start early — around the age of 40. As you can see, there is a clear link between thyroid issues and the menopause.

Let's now examine each menopausal symptom in turn and work out exactly why they happen during this time of your life. Please note, advice for dealing with some of these symptoms will be given in the coming chapters. Consider this your "why" educational chapter, with more to come later on how to deal with these issues.

### Weight Gain

Some women notice that during the menopause they put on weight really easily, and it usually settles around the abdomen and midriff. This is called visceral fat and it is hard to shift once it sets up home. It is also a dangerous type of fat because it settles around the major organs.

Apart from causing health issues, weight gain also affects the way a woman feels about herself, which further compounds the overall effects of the menopause itself. By reducing your weight, you can increase your confidence, looking and feeling great in the process.

I will not dwell too much on this particular problem here, but if you want to learn more, please check my other comprehensive book on this subject, *Beat Your Menopause Weight Gain: Balance Hormones, Stop Middle-Age Spread, Boost Your Health and Vitality*. The book is packed with hints and tips on reducing menopausal weight gain and feeling better about yourself from the inside out. You will learn all about why weight gain happens during the menopause, the hormones that cause it, and what you can do about your menopausal weight gain. The book is available on Amazon.

## *Hot Flushes and Night Sweats*

Two of the most common symptoms of the menopause are, without a doubt, hot flushes and night sweats. Most women will experience these symptoms, although to varying degrees.

A hot flush can be described loosely as a feeling of heat that comes over you quickly and without warning. It starts in one place in the body (varying from person to person), and it spreads very quickly. It often goes as quickly as it comes. Some women might notice that their face becomes flushed at the same time, whilst others may show no outside appearance of feeling hot at all. Some women may also have palpitations at the same time.

Night sweats cause excessive sweating while you are asleep, and you may wake up soaking wet. Many women are forced to change their nightclothes and bedsheets. They are very similar to hot flushes. The main difference is they happen during sleep and they can wake you up. Again, night sweats can disappear as quickly as they came. After the night sweat ends, you might be left freezing cold and in need of an extra blanket.

Hot flushes and night sweats are caused by (surprise, surprise!) hormones. The decline in oestrogen and progesterone has a knock-on effect on the other hormones in the body, especially the thyroid hormones which regulate body temperature. As a result, you may experience these surges and drops in body temperature, before returning to normal.

Both of these issues can be embarrassing, but they can also be rather worrying if you are not sure what is going on. If your hot flushes cause you to have palpitations, you might start to develop anxiety and panic, believing that you are having a heart attack. Of course, you are not, and breathing slowly and deeply should allow your heart rate to return to normal. Women who are experiencing their first few hot flushes, perhaps with palpitations brought on as a result, can experience this worry because they are not sure what is happening. This will also increase their anxiety levels.

### *Mood Changes, Irritation and Anxiety*

Most women will notice a change in their mood occasionally during the menopause. This may be more severe for some women than others. The feeling of wanting to snap at everyone and everything, feeling agitated and annoyed for no reason, and then perhaps feeling extremely down, are quite common.

Again, as with most symptoms, we need to look towards the decreasing level of oestrogen and progesterone within the body. It is very common for this to cause mood changes, depression in some cases, anxiety, and a general lack of energy. As your body adjusts to the lower oestrogen level, this should even itself out. If you are really struggling, do not struggle alone; reach out for help from your doctor and discuss your problems with them.

### Reduced Libido and Vaginal Dryness

The reduction in the two female sex hormones can have a drastic effect on libido for some women. Many women notice that they feel far less bothered about sex during the perimenopausal period in particular.

These dwindling hormones can also lead to vaginal dryness which can cause discomfort and even pain during sex. Of course, this will also have a knock-on effect on how you feel about having intercourse and is likely to place it far down your priority list. This may affect your relationship if you are in one, so you must communicate with your partner and let them know what is going on — they may take it personally and blame themselves for your lack of sexual desire.

### Weak Bones

The menopause changes your body in many different ways, but as you age, you will most probably notice the changes in your body. As oestrogen levels drop, bone density levels drop along with it. This is because oestrogen helps to keep your bones strong, healthy and flexible, and the less oestrogen there is, the more chance you have of weakening bones, placing you at a higher risk of fractures and breaks.

Over time, you may develop a risk of osteoporosis, also known as brittle or weak bones. When this happens, it is far easier to fracture/break a bone than otherwise. However, just because you are going through the menopause, it does not mean this is necessarily going to happen; the risk of osteoporosis increases as you age in general, and there are things you can do to help protect against this. We will talk about that in far more detail as we move through the book, but most of it comes down to simple lifestyle changes and awareness of what a healthy lifestyle involves.

### Changes to the Menstrual Cycle

Every woman experiences this particular symptom while approaching the menopause. By the end of the menopause your symptoms will have stopped completely, but in the years leading up to it, i.e. in the perimenopausal period, you will notice that your periods become irregular in terms of timing and/or flow. They may be lighter or heavier for a while, they will stop and then restart again, and will basically cause you a little bit of inconvenience.

The lowering of the two sex hormones means that your periods are not regular and are not within a pattern like they used to be. It is impossible to predict your periods during the perimenopausal stage because your hormones are playing havoc with them.

### Problems Sleeping

The whole cocktail of problems and hormonal imbalance that the menopause brings can easily disrupt a woman's sleep pattern and make it harder to get a good night's shut eye.

As oestrogen and progesterone decline, hot flushes and night sweats begin, anxiety and low mood may start, can make it very hard to either get to sleep in the first place or stay asleep for long. The more sleep deprived you become, the worse you feel the following day. This is one of the reasons why some menopausal women feel quite tired and drained most of the time.

### Palpitations and Headaches

You may be tired of hearing "it's because of your hormones." However, hormones are responsible for causing the risk of palpitations and headaches.

Palpitations during menopause are often harmless, but you should seek medical help if they are too frequent or you feel worried about them. For the most part, palpitations occur during a hot flush, due to your body temperature surging.

Headaches are also likely to be frequent at this time, again due to hormonal imbalance.

However, if you are worried about your heart palpitations and recurring headaches or migraines, you must check them out with your doctor. There are many other reasons for these symptoms to occur, and they may not be brought on by the menopause only. It is important to do a proper examination if they are very regular or causing you significant discomfort.

### Focus and Concentration Problems

Due to your hormones being in decline, you might experience brain fog during the perimenopausal period. You have no doubt heard about the "baby brain" that new mothers get, which is down to hormones at that time. The same goes for the trouble concentrating that you might experience during the perimenopausal period.

If the menopause keeps affecting your mood significantly, causing you anxiety and depression, that could also be the reason for your focus and concentration issues.

### Increased Frequency of UTIs

As this is one of the less common menopausal symptoms, I will not allocate a chapter to this particular issue, but it is worth discussing it briefly in this section. UTIs (urinary tract infections) or water infections, as they are more commonly known, may become more frequent during the menopause for some women. Again, this is down to oestrogen levels declining.

As oestrogen declines, the urethra changes a little. This is the tube that takes urine from the bladder and outside as you urinate. It depends how this decreased oestrogen level affects your particular urethra, but for some women this can be enough to lead to a higher risk of UTIs. They are not particularly pleasant, as you will know if you have ever had one. Most importantly, they can easily be treated by your doctor.

In this chapter, I have highlighted the most common menopausal symptoms, along with a quick rundown of why they are likely to be happening to you. You will notice one very clear pattern in all of them, which is a decrease in female sex hormones as the primary cause.

This is the main reason for all menopausal symptoms occurring, and the power those hormones have over your entire body can be quite startling if you are not informed of what is going on. Now you know exactly the reason for your symptoms, and that should give you a certain amount of reassurance that you are going through an entirely normal process called the menopause. However, as I have mentioned a few times already, if you are at all worried, I advise you to speak to your doctor for reassurance, and further advice by doing some tests and getting to the bottom of your troublesome symptoms.

# Key Points

- Every woman is unique and might experience different menopausal symptoms from those of their friends or family members.

- There are several common menopausal symptoms. However, the most common include hot flushes, night sweats, weight gain, mood changes, anxiety, vaginal dryness and low libido, bone weakness, sleep issues, and problems concentrating.

- It is important to get familiar with the most common menopausal symptoms and understand why they occur.

- Hot flushes and night sweats are the most complained about menopausal symptoms, and these can also cause issues with sleep.

- Changing your lifestyle can help with many menopausal symptoms.

- If you are not sure if a symptom you experience is harmless or not, or if you are struggling with the severity of your symptoms, visit your doctor. You should always check things out if something is troubling you and causing you discomfort.

# Chapter 3

# A Word About HRT

Most women who go to see their doctor about menopausal symptoms are given the option of hormone replacement therapy (HRT). Some women are totally against it, others are open to it, and some of them are not quite sure. It is important to get as much information on the subject as possible before deciding whether this is the right treatment for you.

HRT is not a blanket approach to the menopause. You do not have to take it, you might not even need to take it, perhaps you are not suitable for it, but many women are offered it. It is essential to know the facts about HRT and make an informed choice that is personal to you.

There are many benefits to taking HRT, but there are also some side effects and risks. If you choose not to go with HRT, there are a few alternative options that you may want to consider. This will be discussed later on in this chapter.

Because HRT is a standard menopausal treatment and your doctor is likely to offer it to you for treating your symptoms, an entire chapter in this book is dedicated to this subject to give you the necessary information that you need to know.

HRT is given as a medical treatment to women going through the menopause (if they choose to take it) to help relieve the menopausal symptoms. As the name suggests, the drug replaces some of the hormones that have been reduced due to the menopause. If a woman is having an incredibly hard time with one or more symptoms, HRT may help to relieve them.

Most women can take HRT, but as with anything, there are a few anomalies. You might not be able to take HRT if you have any history or a family history of breast, ovarian or endometrial cancer, blood clots, or if you have liver disease or any problems with high blood pressure (hypertension). If you do have blood pressure problems, your doctor will need to stabilise it with medication before considering whether to prescribe HRT. Always listen to your doctor's advice on suitability and be sure to consider your decision very carefully. You do not have to make a decision immediately; you can go away and think about it first.

## The Benefits and Side Effects of HRT

The main benefit of HRT is that it can reduce troublesome menopausal symptoms and therefore allow you to go through the menopause with far less trouble. This does not mean that you will not have any symptoms at all, but they will be far fewer and more manageable.

It is still a good idea to make lifestyle changes if you are taking HRT, because focusing on your overall health and well-being by following a healthy diet, doing regular exercise and establishing a healthy sleep routine as you become a little older is always recommendable regardless. This will also help you to become more mindful of what constitutes positive and healthy versus what does not. It is easy to fall into unhealthy patterns and habits as we go through life, so this is an excellent opportunity to look at the rights and wrongs and readjust.

HRT has always had a slightly dubious reputation. This is because, whilst it is a very effective treatment for many women, it does have a few risks attached to it. The benefits are often thought to outweigh the downsides, but it is something that has to be decided on carefully if you are interested in trying this drug. I recommend you speak to your doctor, who will weigh up the pros and cons with you and find the best type for you (more on that shortly) and ultimately decide whether or not it is safe for you.

The main side effects of HRT include:

- Tender breasts

- Headaches

- Nausea

- Indigestion

- Bloating

- Vaginal bleeding

- Abdominal pain

- Leg cramps

If you do experience side effects when taking HRT, they are usually mild and they should even out after about three months of taking them. However, if you find the side effects too troublesome or they are worrying you, go to see your doctor and change the type you are taking or ask the doctor for an alternative. Remember, just because you are going through the menopause, does not mean that you have to take HRT. It is an option that is there for you if you want it.

If you do decide to take HRT, there is not an actual time frame on how long you can take it for, but your doctor will advise you on when you should stop.

Most women stop taking HRT after their menopausal symptoms have settled down. There is an increased risk of breast cancer linked to HRT, so this is something you have to bear in mind when it comes to deciding whether to start taking it and how long to take it for. You can choose to stop taking HRT whenever you want to, but it is a good idea to wean yourself off to check whether or not your menopause symptoms come back. If they do, you can continue taking it for a bit longer.

## Different Types of HRT

There are a few different types of HRT, and your doctor will advise you on the best one for you.

Here are the main types:

- *Combination* – e.g. a combination of both oestrogen and progesterone, to replace what you are naturally lacking. This can be done through tablets, skin patches, gels, pessaries, rings, or a vaginal cream.

- *Oestrogen-only* – Women who have had a hysterectomy in the past, e.g. no longer have a womb, can take oestrogen only HRT, and again, this is available in different formats, such as tablets, gels, etc.

There are different ways to take HRT. You might start on a lower dose, and then it might get increased at the later stage. You may even be prescribed to take oestrogen continually and then progesterone added in for a few weeks and then repeat the cycle; it depends on your body and what it needs. Your doctor will advise you about this.

## Possible Alternatives to HRT

Of course, you might not want to take HRT and that is fine. There are a few alternatives you could look into and again, it is up to you whether you go with them or not.

Many women stick to lifestyle changes only and it works very well for them. We are all different, so make sure you choose a method of working your way through the menopause that suits you and your needs. Your friend might swear by one particular method, but you might try it and find no relief whatsoever.

The main alternatives to HRT, aside from lifestyle changes alone, include:

- Tibolone

- Antidepressants

- Clonidine

- Complementary therapies

## *Tibolone*

You will find Tibolone marketed under the name "Livial" and this is a drug that your doctor has to prescribe. Tibolone is similar to HRT in that it puts back the hormones you are lacking, and it is thought to be particularly useful for hot flushes, mood problems, and reduced libido in particular.

Only postmenopausal women can take Tibolone and it is designed to help with the dwindling menopausal symptoms as they can last for many years after the menopause is established. There are side effects (abdominal and pelvic pain, tender breasts, vaginal discharge and itching) and there is an increased risk of breast cancer and strokes, so discuss this option carefully with your doctor beforehand.

## *Antidepressants*

Some women find that antidepressants can help them with their menopausal symptoms, especially hot flushes and low mood. Whilst antidepressants are not licensed for menopausal symptom use, they are thought to be useful, so it is up to you to look at this possibility.

We all know that antidepressants can have some unpleasant side effects, such as agitation, nausea, reduced libido, dizziness, and anxiety. These side effects usually reduce and disappear after three months of use but again, you need to discuss this with your doctor if you are struggling.

## *Clonidine*

Clonidine is used for treating high blood pressure, drug withdrawal, and attention deficit hyperactivity disorder (ADHD).

For women struggling with hot flushes and night sweats, in particular, Clonidine could be very useful. As Clonidine is not associated with hormones, there is no increased risk of breast cancer to consider, and this appeals to many women. However, some women may not find this medication very effective for their menopausal symptoms.

Clonidine usually takes around two weeks to a month to show significant effects and can cause tiredness, constipation, dry mouth, and even depression. Again, speak to your doctor if you think Clonidine might help you, or you are struggling with its side effects.

## *Alternative Medicine*

I want to point out that most alternative medicines are not backed up by scientific evidence, yet many women do try them, so I want to put a few ideas here for you to consider for yourself.

You will find a few products on the shelves of health stores or online that are reputed to help with specific menopausal symptoms, the main ones being:

- Evening primrose oil

- St John's wort

- Ginseng

- Black cohosh

- Angelica

Most of these are reputed to reduce hot flushes in particular, but the problem is that the complementary and alternative industry is not regulated in the same way as the pharmaceutical industry. That means you can purchase a product believing it is high-quality, but the ingredients either are not good quality, or you are not recommended to take the right dose. I will not give you recommendations on which companies are the best sources of high-quality products, as it depends on what is suitable in the country you reside in, but I suggest you do your research on this.

When searching on the internet, it is worth mentioning that it is a good idea to spend a little more money and find a quality product with plenty of positive reviews, rather than opting for a lower cost one. Please note that taking a supplement with the brand name does not mean it is a good quality supplement. It is also important to remember that when taking a cheap supplement, you often get what you pay for.

This chapter has given you a few ideas on how you might like to treat your menopausal symptoms medically. But you do not have to do this, and you might prefer to stay with natural methods via changing your diet and adding in a few healthy lifestyle measures. The choice is yours, but it is essential to look at different options when searching for the best solution. It is vital to get the information you need from reliable sources to choose how to approach your menopausal journey based on your own informed decision.

The rest of this book focuses on managing menopausal symptoms naturally instead of using supplements or medications. Dealing with my menopausal symptoms naturally was my preferred way and when my doctor offered me HRT, I refused to take it.

Prioritising a healthy lifestyle will affect your hormones and make a positive difference in your life as a menopausal woman. You can do many things to help yourself, and there are numerous methods you can apply to help you live a healthy and symptom-free life.

# Key Points

- HRT stands for hormone replacement therapy, and it replaces hormones that are at a lower level due to approaching the menopause.

- Not all women use HRT, but it is an option for you if you want to take it.

- There are benefits to taking HRT, but there are also side effects and these need to be discussed with your doctor and weighed up.

- The final decision over whether you take HRT or not is yours, but it is not suitable for some women and your doctor will inform you if you fall into that category.

- HRT does not completely take away your menopausal symptoms, but it may help reduce their severity, therefore making the menopause more manageable for you.

- Some of the most common HRT side effects include tender breasts, headaches, nausea, indigestion, abdominal pain and vaginal bleeding.

- There are several types of HRT and a few alternatives to explore with your doctor.

- Alternative medicine should be discussed with your doctor before you consider using them.

# Chapter 4

# Battling Hot Flushes and Night Sweats

As I have already mentioned, two of the most common menopausal symptoms that affect most women at this time of life are hot flushes and night sweats. Hot flushes, in particular, are incredibly annoying, can feel embarrassing and uncomfortable, and they tend to come out of nowhere.

On the other hand, night sweats can cause many health issues as they prevent you from having a good night's sleep. Lack of sleep can negatively impact your health causing you to have a low mood, increased irritability, and difficulty concentrating. It can also affect your appetite, which could lead you towards putting on weight.

You will quickly come to see that most symptoms affect one another.

In an earlier chapter of this book, I talked about the fact that hot flushes and night sweats are both caused by an imbalance of hormones, affecting the thyroid, which regulates body temperature. A few of the treatment methods I talked about in the last chapter can be very useful for hot flushes in particular, but even if you go down the medical route, e.g. HRT or one of the alternatives I mentioned, you are likely to need to make a few changes to your routine too. Handily, it is relatively easy to do it once you know how, and the effects can be far-reaching.

# Lifestyle Changes to Reduce Hot Flushes and Night Sweats

There are a few things you can do to reduce hot flushes and night sweats, and it is not impossible to eliminate them completely. Soon we will look at the importance of a healthy diet and how it links to this particular symptom. First, let us focus on to general changes you can make to your lifestyle and routine so that these symptoms become a fleeting issue rather than a chronic problem that stays with you for a long time and makes you feel miserable.

### *Wear Light Clothing*

You need to be warm if it is sub-zero outside, but when you are in the house or at work, try wearing light clothing if possible, and avoid synthetic materials that hold in the heat and make you feel a little sweaty. Lightweight cotton is an excellent fabric to keep you cool.

When you go to bed, choose only light clothing and think about breathable materials for your bedding too. The more cool air that can move around you, the more comfortable you will feel. Sure, this will not stop you from having these symptoms, but it will reduce their severity and help make you more comfortable in general. When a hot flush arrives, it will not be as burning hot, and after experiencing night sweats you might have less of a clammy feeling. These changes and improvements can be quite dramatic when you make the right adjustments.

### Regulate the Bedroom Temperature

If night sweats are a big problem for you, regulating your bedroom temperature could help. Keep your bedroom as cool as you can, perhaps opening windows and using a fan to circulate air around the room. As before, stick to light and breathable fabrics for whatever you wear for bed and for the bedding itself. If you have air conditioning in your room, make use of it and set it on a moderate temperature.

This change can be difficult if your partner likes the room a little warmer, but you are going to have to have a conversation in that case and make them understand your position. There is bound to be some middle ground you can arrive at and if you are waking them up because you are bothered by hot flushes and night sweats, they might welcome this adjustment because it means they get a better night's sleep.

### Sip on Cold Drinks

You might love tea and coffee, but drinking hot drinks will send your temperature up, and when this is already a problem, it will not help you.

Keep a jug of water or juice in the fridge filled with ice cubes and regularly sip on it. Or use an insulated mug to keep the contents chilled. By doing that, you are helping to keep your body temperature down and helping reduce hot flushes throughout the day. You are also staying hydrated, which is very important for overall health and well-being and will have a related effect on other troublesome symptoms, such as headaches.

### Stop Smoking

Smoking is damaging for your health in general, but it could be making your hot flushes much worse. Studies suggest that quitting smoking decreases the risk of midlife hot flushes and showed that smoking could reduce oestrogen levels in the body, therefore increasing your risk of having a hot flush. This means that the more you smoke, the worse your flushes will be.

Make a healthy choice to stop smoking for the sake of your health, but also to reduce your hot flushes. The benefits of quitting smoking are tremendous for health and general well-being. If you need help to stop smoking, discuss this with your doctor, who may be able to refer you to a smoking cessation advisor. There are many methods that can help you quit smoking, including patches, meditation, and good old willpower. Whatever method you choose, quitting smoking will prove to be one of the best decisions you will ever make and will certainly affect many of the other symptoms you may be experiencing, in a very positive way.

### Exercise Regularly

I am sure you are aware that exercise is good for your health. Exercising regularly is vital for your heart health, mood, and gives a myriad of other great benefits. But did you know that exercise might also help to reduce the severity and intensity of your hot flushes?

Studies show that exercising can benefit menopausal symptoms and the study done by Harvard medical school showed a 60% reduction in the frequency of hot flushes after experiencing an increased heart rate due to exercising.

I know that many women are familiar with the countless benefits of exercise, but did you know that doing too much exercise can be as bad for you as leading a sedentary lifestyle. "Why is this?" you may ask.

As I mentioned earlier, menopause decreases oestrogen levels, which is one of the main reasons for your hot flushes. Excess exercise can further lower your oestrogen. Also, too much exercise could put your body under stress which will increase your cortisol levels. Cortisol is a stress hormone and known to cause hot flushes. I suggest you look at the type of exercise you choose to do and the level you are going to perform your aerobic activity.

Moderation is the key, remember this. You do not need to pound the treadmill at the gym every single day; you simply need to get your heart rate up and sweat a little (ironic, right?). Your body will naturally regulate its own temperature, which will eliminate those irregularities.

By doing this, not only will you become fitter and healthier and your mood will improve, but you will also find that you have fewer hot flushes. Combining this with the other methods I have mentioned will give you a greater chance of success and help with a range of other symptoms that we are going to look at throughout the rest of the book.

### *Reduce Your Stress Levels*

Stress is no good for your health, and it is one of the leading killers in today's society. Not only can it worsen your hot flushes and night sweats, but it can also prove to be fatal for your health when allowed to accumulate over a more extended period. It might sound drastic, but it is true. The more stress you allow into your life, the more cortisol your body will produce. Over a long period of time, this can lead to having far too much cortisol circulating around your body.

Cortisol is a stress hormone. When the raised cortisol level interacts with your female sex-hormones which are imbalanced due to the menopause, your hot flushes are likely to be more troublesome than ever before, along with an impending sense of doom and anxiety that stress tends to initiate.

Reducing stress is not easy, but there are ways you can do it. Try meditation, play a sport or exercise, focus on sleep and diet, and talk about whatever is bothering you. We tend to hold everything inside and allow stress to build and build, until we reach the point of no return.

Allowing stress to take over your life is no good for your health and it is no good for your hot flushes or night sweats either.

Stress management is a very real thing, so make sure you pay attention to changing your routine and make it a priority.

# The Role of Diet

What you eat can affect your hot flushes and night sweats too. Certain foods are good for you and could have a beneficial effect on reducing the number of hot flushes and night sweats you are experiencing, and there are some which are best to avoid.

When you eat highly processed foods, rich in sugar or salt and unhealthy fats, then chemicals and hormones in your body change. This affects your menopausal symptoms and can increase the frequency and strength of the hot flushes you experience.

To prove the importance of a good diet with women experiencing hot flushes, a study done by medical anthropologist Margaret Lock in 1998 found that Japanese women suffered less hot flushes than women in the western world. This is thought to be down to a different kind of diet, which focuses more on fresh and clean foods, as opposed to the western-style diet rich in processed foods, high sugar content, and many synthetic ingredients.

Convenience foods were invented to help keep us sane and afloat in an increasingly busy world, but if we consider the toll it takes on our health, both physical and mental, it turns out they are far from convenient. I understand that if you rarely cook food from scratch, the prospect of doing so regularly could be intimidating. But the more time you practice this skill, the more you handle vegetables, roots, and grains in their original forms, the more comfortable you will get with them.

If you want to reduce your hot flushes and night sweats, be sure to eat more of the foods on the "do" list and less of the ones on the "do not" list below.

*Do list:*

- *Fresh fruit and vegetables* – Not only are these far better for your health, but many researchers have found that a Mediterranean-style diet, i.e. a diet which is packed with fresh, whole foods, can help to reduce the number of hot flushes a woman experiences. Every additional serving of whole, nutrient-dense plants will have a positive impact on your health.

- *Whole-grains* – Again, these are a much healthier alternative to processed grains that can increase hot flushes and cause all manner of digestive issues. Stick to whole-grain versions of bread, rice, pasta, etc.

- *Soy* – There is some suggestion that soy products, such as soy milk, edamame beans and tofu, could help to reduce the number of hot flushes and night sweats a woman experiences in menopause. It is because the oestrogen from plants can regulate the hormones in your body and therefore reduce your symptoms as a result.

- *Flax seeds* – Flax seeds contain the healthy types of fat you need in your diet for overall health and well-being, and you can easily sprinkle these onto your morning porridge or your muesli, or just throw them into something you are baking. They are rich in plant oestrogen and they can balance hormone levels and drastically cut the number of hot flushes in many cases.

- **Strawberries** – Not only are they delicious, but strawberries are thought to reduce hot flushes. Again, it is down to the fact that they contain plant oestrogen. Besides, they are also high in Vitamin C, giving you an immune system boost and balancing out your hormones.

- **Healthy fats** – I have already mentioned flax seeds, but the healthy type of fat is an excellent addition to your diet if you want to reduce hot flushes and increase your general health and well-being. Omega-3 fatty acids are the best type to focus on here, and that means a good weekly intake of fatty fish, such as mackerel, sardines, etc. You can also get a fair amount of omega-3 fatty acids from leafy green vegetables, canola oil and soybeans.

### Do not list:

- **Spicy foods** – Any food which causes your body temperature to rise is likely to bring on a hot flush, and foods that are high in spice content do exactly this. Avoid chillies as they contain capsaicin which dilates blood vessels and increases temperature. Black pepper contains piperine, which does the same thing.

- *Alcohol* – Of course, everything in moderation, but alcohol is known to increase hot flushes for many women. Again, it dilates the blood vessels and makes hot flushes more likely. This does not happen to all women, but it is a fairly common effect. If you love your evening glass of wine, I suggest that you cut down and have it less frequently, or find an alcoholic beverage that affects you less.

- *Caffeine* – Opt for decaffeinated drinks rather than the full-on caffeinated versions as caffeine can make hot flushes worse. If you really cannot do without, try and let your coffee cool down before drinking it and limit your intake to one cup per day.

- *Sugar* – Many studies have found that women who have a high sugar diet tend to have more hot flushes. In that case, you need to cut down as much as you can, and of course, that will also help your overall health. It is recommended by WHO (World Health Organisation) that you should consume less than six teaspoons of sugar every day, so that is a good marker to aim for. If you have a sweet tooth, you might find this a tough habit to kick but try substituting your sweet treats for other healthier options, such as yogurt, fruit, and nuts. It can be done!

If you have not done it already, I advise you to visit bit.ly/menopause-healthy-recipes-1 and download *Healthy*

*Eating for Menopause – Recipe Book*. It is packed with delicious recipes to support you on your menopause journey.

By making the right kind of lifestyle changes and watching what you eat, you might be able to reduce your hot flushes and night sweats down to a minimum; in some cases, you may be able to rid yourself of them completely. Just remember, by the time you are 50, you will have eaten more than 50,000 meals. That is a considerable tradition to contend with, so have patience with yourself. Start with one step at a time.

### My Client Ronnie

I want to tell you about my client, Ronnie (the name has been changed, to respect the privacy of my client). When I first met her, she had just turned 50. Not only was she trying to overcome her weight loss issues, but fluctuations of hormones during the menopause also starting to overwhelm her.

Sleepless nights had never bothered her in the past, but the missing sleep suddenly made her days feel never-ending and an uphill battle. She used to have regular night sweats which kept her awake most nights. Even though she was constantly exhausted, she still could not sleep. This was an extremely frustrating experience for her.

She also struggled with hot flushes during the day. They did not help her comfort levels at all. In the most inopportune moments, she would overheat, leaving her soaked through with sweat in minutes. She found this unbearable at times.

Many women struggle with this experience, and there is nothing that can prepare us for it. But it is important to know that simple diet and lifestyle changes can often reduce the frequency and severity of these symptoms of menopause.

With plenty of encouragement and support, Ronnie made a few changes to her nutrition and the way she was eating. She also followed my advice on getting into habit of moving her body more often. Within a month, she was sleeping soundly enough to feel rested most days and when I asked her about her hot flushes, she could not even remember the last time she had them.

What she was really excited about, however, was the fact that she not only enjoyed her new, healthy meal plan, but she did not feel like she was on a diet. She was never hungry. Also, she was losing weight.

By focusing on her health, Ronnie was able to naturally help her body address the issues so many women struggle with — disordered eating and weight management. And she was learning to love her body in her early fifties because she had an entirely new lease on life that was completely unexpected.

## Key Points

- Hot flushes and night sweats are the most common symptom with menopausal women, and they can be very annoying and upsetting.

- Hot flushes, in particular, can come and go quickly or stick around for longer.

- Hot flushes and night sweats can affect your sleep pattern and therefore make many of your other menopausal symptoms worse.

- Wear light clothing to bed and make sure your room temperature is not too hot.

- Smoking can make hot flushes worse, so work on quitting smoking to improve your general health and well-being.

- Regular exercise can reduce instances of hot flushes.

- Stress can also make hot flushes worse, so work on stress management.

- Diet plays a role in hot flushes, and there are several foods you should focus on and avoid to help hot flushes becoming a significant problem for you.

# Chapter 5

# The Mental Health Effects of the Menopause

The menopause does not just affect your body, but your mind too. Changes in your hormones can throw your emotions for a much unexpected turn and you may experience low mood, agitation, anxiety, stress, mood swings and low confidence.

While we would never say that it is "normal" to feel this way, some people would argue that it is normal for the menopause to be this way. Feeling depressed, anxious, agitated, etc. is often a result of the hormonal imbalance that is in charge of a woman's body during the menopause transition. Some women might feel that something far more worrying is going on when they experience these symptoms, but I can assure you that it is the hormones that affect your well-being. That is the power that hormones can have over you.

Nowadays, we are increasingly encouraged to talk about our mental health, which can only be a good thing. Almost everyone will experience low mood at some point in their lives, and if you have experienced this once or twice already, you will know that it is not something you will want to put up with. The truth is that you DO NOT have to just put up with feeling this way and there is plenty you can do to help yourself, or you can reach out and get help from others.

During this time of your life, seeking help to support your emotional and psychological needs might be necessary. This can be done in many different ways and some women choose to take supplements or medication, while others decide to go to talking therapies or join activities such as yoga or meditation.

Do not feel that because you are going through the menopause you simply have to just deal with the symptoms that are common for this time in a woman's life. Not doing anything about it is a fast track to a miserable menopause, which may go on for many years. I suggest you be proactive and work on making your life more comfortable. Remember, you are in the driving seat. You have to decide where you are going and make sure that you get there safely.

In the following sections, I will give you many suggestions and plenty of guidance on the actions you can take to feel good about your body, and be positive about your life, so that the menopause will feel more like a light breeze rather than a hurricane blowing in your face at a speed of 150 miles per hour.

## You Do Not Have to Suffer From Low Mood

The hormonal imbalance caused by the perimenopause and menopause itself can cause chaos on so many levels, but the effects can be the hardest to deal with as far as mental health is concerned. It is essential to talk to your family and friends as much as possible because perhaps they do not realise how you are feeling, and they do not understand why you might occasionally snap at them. They want to help and support you, but first, you need to open up and talk about how you are feeling. Having them on your side will certainly make things easier and will also reduce the chances of fallouts and arguments.

In the past, women have assumed that experiencing low mood, having difficulty concentrating and focusing, or suffering from anxiety, stress, and mood swings is something that is expected of middle-age women. But we do not live in those days anymore. Nowadays, we do not have to bear the symptoms of the menopause and there are lots of things we can do to reduce the severity of the symptoms.

Poor mental health can be caused by so many things, including the menopause, but not one of these causes is a good enough reason for feeling low or agitated or being constantly anxious. We talk so openly about our physical health, but we are still worried about opening up too much about our mental health. Why not make a pact with yourself that one good thing to come out of the menopause for you will be an openness about how you are feeling, a willingness to talk about things that upset you, and focusing on self-care? I think we could all do with more of that, whether we are going through the menopause or not.

Of course, the changes your body is going through can cause you to feel less confident, but remember that you are not less of a woman or less attractive because you are going through the menopause. You are not less worthy than before because of the changes you are going through, and not one stage of the menopause defines you as a woman. This can be difficult to accept when you are going through it, however that is where focusing on self-care comes into it. In many ways, when done in the right way, the menopause can increase your confidence, believe it or not. You will finally understand your body and your power as a woman.

The more you focus on looking after yourself; the mind, body, and soul, the more you will notice your self-confidence increasing. Also, the more you practice gratitude, the happier and healthier you will be — inside and out. New opportunities will come your way as a result of it all, and who knows where those new chances in life may take you.

# How to Naturally Boost Your Feel-Good Factor

There are many ways you can practice self-care and make yourself feel better in the process. I am going to share some techniques with you that you can try without making a huge effort, but the effects will be substantial.

Many women feel that they do not deserve a little pampering and the time to focus on themselves. Some women feel guilty about having "me time". They feel as though they are being selfish because they are so used to dedicating their time and love to everyone else around them. It almost seems "wrong" to focus on themselves every now and then.

Here are some suggestions to help you give yourself a break and focus on your own needs instead of pleasing everybody else, i.e. your spouse, children, elderly parents, work colleagues, friends, etc. This is YOUR time and you need it — you deserve it!

### Be Kind to Yourself

Be kind to yourself is my first suggestion. You are going through a change in your life and any change is sure to make you feel a little out of sorts. Make peace with that fact and accept that it is perfectly acceptable to feel that way.

Far too often women have been forced to simply "get on with it" as quietly as possible, but we are not in the 1800s anymore! We are allowed to talk about how we are feeling and make time for ourselves.

Self-care is vital during this time in your life. Be kind to yourself and do the things that make you happy. If you love to spend time having a warm bubble bath before bedtime or read a book, then do it. If you love going to the cinema and eating a bucket of popcorn to yourself, why not do it? (Occasionally, of course). If dancing is your thing, grab your dancing shoes! Whatever makes you feel good and gives you confidence, you need to do more of it, and take the time to really nourish your mind, body, and soul.

Everything in moderation should be your mantra. So, if you fancy having a piece of cake once per week, then do it. Moderation is key and will unlock the door to health and happiness. One piece of chocolate cake a week is not going to kill you, and one session in the gym with a personal trainer will not make you fit, slim and healthy. Distinguishing what is healthy and what is unhealthy for you is the key. And creating the balance using this knowledge is crucial.

### Practice Positivity

I often hear women having a conversation with one another and discussing how the menopause is affecting their physical, mental and emotional state. I also hear them agree that it is normal for menopausal women to be overweight and suffer from countless symptoms that this stage of life can bring. Often, I see the pattern occurring where women feed each other with negativity, creating even more anxiety and low mood.

I can assure you that it is entirely possible to boost your mood and help you feel more in control of your body and mind by learning to become more positive. Of course, this takes time and you need to expect results to come to you cumulatively and not overnight. Whilst positivity will not automatically remove your troubles and worries, it will allow you to cope with them in much healthier and more productive ways. You will start to see challenges as learning curves, rather than instantly being laid low by them. This can be extremely useful during the menopause, when challenges may come your way on a regular basis.

There are many ways to practice positivity and I want to mention two techniques, that are particularly useful for helping you to see the glass as half full instead of half empty. They are called positive affirmation and reframing. Applying these two methods will have far-reaching benefits on your life as they will open your mind to the opportunities around you, and who knows where they may lead?

### *Method Number One – Positive Affirmations*

Affirmations are positive statements that you keep repeating to yourself. It is a powerful activity which can help you change the way you think and remove negative language that you have a habit of using when talking to yourself. This technique can help you to become more positive and overcome your negative thinking and behaviours. It has been proven that the repetition of statements can positively affect your conscious and unconscious mind.

Here are 15 affirmations that can change your state of mind and help you stay positive. Repeat them out loud several times a day and focus on their meaning. Early morning and before bedtime are two the best times for this. At first you might find it a little strange, but the more you do it, the more you will feel confident doing it. Watch your thoughts during this activity, believe your words, and they will become real.

- I am strong

- I am positive

- I am unique

- I am powerful

- I am fearless

- I am attractive

- I am confident

- I am smart

- I love my body

- I fully accept myself

- I am proud of myself

- I truly love myself

- I am grateful for everything I have

- I am who I want to be

- I am enough

***Method Number Two – Reframing***

Another powerful method for practising positivity is called reframing. It is a type of cognitive behavioural therapy technique that replaces a negative thought with a positive one. This technique helps you to become more aware of your self-talk and the effects it has on you.

Here is how it might work in practice:

- You have a negative thought and you acknowledge it as negative, e.g. "I have lines under my eyes, and I hate them".

- You take this negative thought and turn it into something positive, e.g. "I have lines under my eyes, which show my wisdom and experience".

- You would then repeat this new thought several times, and every time you notice the lines under your eyes you would repeat it again.

- Repetition is critical here because, over time, your brain will think of the positive thought, before the negative one and assume that to be true.

The more you reframe negative thoughts that pop into your mind, the more you will become a generally more positive person overall.

A combination of doing positive affirmation and practising reframing can significantly impact the way you feel about yourself and the direction your life is going to take.

Give it a try! It is very easy to apply them in your everyday life.

They will enhance your life not just in overcoming the negative mental health effects of the menopause but also helping you be a more positive person. This will improve your relationship with others and help you to be much kinder to yourself.

**Meditation and Mindfulness**

Many women find that practising mindfulness can help them to feel happier and more uplifted. Adopting mindfulness in your life will allow you to be present and live in the moment, rather than thinking about the past, or jumping ahead and worrying about the future.

If you find meditation difficult at first, persevere. It is hard to quieten your mind when you have been so used to all the noise around you, but you can develop it with time. Mindfulness meditation is often easier than regular meditation because you can do it on the go. All you need to do is be aware of what is around you. So, the next time you are out walking, avoid looking at your phone and instead tune into your surroundings.

First, calm your mind by focusing on your breathing. Notice the inhaling and exhaling, and keep it controlled and slow. When you are ready, start to observe your surroundings; look at the leaves and how they shine in the light, watch the playful dog running in the field, and see how the clouds move slowly in the sky. The more tuned you are to the present, the more you will be able to simply observe your troubles rather than feel like you need to do something about them, e.g. react emotionally. As thoughts enter your mind, simply acknowledge them but do not overthink it; allow them to float back out and return at a later time, when you are more concerned with them. With practice, this all becomes much easier.

Just as being positive can help you live in a more upbeat and happier way, mindfulness can help you deal with upheaval more effectively and improve your mood. You will start to see the menopause as something that is simply happening to you, not as something which defines you or changes your future. As a result, you will not obsess or worry over small changes, and you will not allow your confidence to be ruined.

### Rest When You Need to

A lot is going on inside your body right now and this means you might feel tired from time to time or even experience fatigue. This is a common complaint from menopausal women, and it is further compounded if you are already struggling to get a good night's sleep.

If you are suffering from fatigue, be kind to yourself and rest whenever you need to. Give yourself permission to listen to your body and make sure you slow down. We all need a little downtime; in fact, it should be on prescription!

Far too many women feel like they have to take on the world and win every single time, but this is an unrealistic expectation and it is not healthy either. Putting too much expectation on yourself will lead to burn out.

Take the time to slow down and focus on doing what your body is asking you to do. You are not failing, you are simply doing what your body needs. As Jim Rohn said "Take care of your body. It is the only place you have to live".

At the moment, your body is dealing with changes and your hormones are fluctuating, some days you might need more rest than others. Simply monitor how you feel on a daily basis and change your routine accordingly. If you feel like everything is on top of you and there is a to-do list as long as your arm to complete, work through it slowly and methodically. Similarly, if you feel you need to take a moment, take it. Listen to your body and let "how you feel" be your guide.

### Regular Exercise

There are several chemicals released in the body during exercise. Some of these are dopamine, serotonin and endorphins. They are brain chemicals that create happy feelings and are known to lift the mood. Exercise can help you feel more upbeat and positive, and as you already learnt, it can be great for controlling hot flushes too. As you can see, there are many benefits from just getting your body moving a little bit more. And if you can incorporate outdoor exercise with fresh air at the same time, you will notice even more benefits.

The healing effects of Mother Nature are ideal for helping to banish worries and relieve stress.

If you have a friend who also wants to exercise more, why not head out together? You will get a social boost, and you will be exercising at the same time.

### Eat Nourishing, Healthy Foods

Eating a healthy diet is beneficial on many different levels, but certain foods can give you the feel-good factor and boost your mood, while others you should try and avoid. You might love a glass of wine in the evening, but you need to proceed with caution. Alcohol is a depressant, and more than one glass could easily tip you towards the lower end of the scale.

Reducing caffeine intake would also be beneficial, as caffeine is a stimulant that can cause anxiety for anyone prone to it.

Here is what you should eat to boost your mood:

- Fatty types of fish, full of healthy omega-3 fatty acids, such as sardines, mackerel, etc.

- Dark chocolate – in moderation!

- Bananas

- Oats

- Fermented foods such as kefir and sauerkraut

- Berries

- Nuts

- Seeds

These super healthy foods are known to help with depression, stabilise your blood sugar levels and improve your mood, and increase feel-good chemicals in your brain and your gut. You can easily incorporate them into your diet. Try to experiment with different recipes and learn new and exciting ways to prepare your meals. It is far easier than you think to pack several healthy ingredients into one meal; you simply need to think creatively and be mindful of what you need in your daily diet.

I strongly suggest you cook your meals rather than relying on fast-food and processed foods. Processed foods will not help your menopausal symptoms. In fact, they are widely known to encourage your symptoms to get much worse.

Some of my clients find it very therapeutic to cook their meals from scratch. It is about being creative and making something from basics with their hands. Creativity and cooking together are known to boost the feel-good factor and help with improving your mood. When you add in the ingredients that are also linked to mood improvement, you are onto a good thing.

One of my clients did exactly that – she started experimenting with new recipes and cooking meals from scratch using fresh ingredients. She was very obese and unhealthy when we began working together. She felt uncomfortable about her physical appearance and was struggling with her self-worth. Then, everything changed!

She started to cook healthy recipes with her two daughters. Spending time with them and cooking healthy meals twice a week brought so much enjoyment to her. The whole family benefited from this experience. My client developed a much closer relationship with her teenage daughters. Also, enjoying healthy foods and eating meals together had a positive effect on the health of the whole family.

If you have not already downloaded a *Healthy Eating for Menopause – Recipe Book*, please visit bit.ly/menopause-healthy-recipes-1 and download your free copy. You will find plenty of delicious recipes there.

### Try Yoga

Yoga teaches you to control your breathing and use it as a grounding tool. Whenever you are feeling stressed, tired, or upset, you can go back to your breathing and slow things down. This is a very calming and healthy way to control stress and anxiety. Yoga has been shown to improve mood, but it could also help strengthen the body and reduce the chances of muscle loss, which could lead to osteoporosis in later life. By incorporating yoga into your daily life, you are giving yourself a tool you can use whenever you feel stressed, upset, angry, tired, or experience any other negative emotion.

Yoga does not have to be about being super-flexible, and there are many different positions you can try that allow you to start from the bottom and work your way up. If you have any problems with your back or another part of the body, you can simply tell the instructor and they will show you a way to perform the yoga pose without aggravating your pre-existing problem.

### Allow Yourself a Social Life

At the end of a long working day, you might feel like hiding away, and when you are feeling a little low in mood, that is most probably what you feel like doing. However, hiding away is not going to make you feel better, and it is likely to further worsen your low mood and anxiety.

There is strength in friendship and even if you are just going to your friend's house for a cup of tea, or you are going out for a meal, make sure you create time for a social life. This is not being indulgent, and it is not a waste of money; it is a vital part of your overall health and well-being and as far as your mental health is concerned, it is crucial. However, there are limits and if you are always out drinking and partying, or maybe you are heading out for food a lot, you might want to rein things in a little and question why you are spending all your spare time and attention in that direction. Remember, everything in moderation.

### Find Support from Other Women

A great way to feel stronger within yourself is to surround yourself with equally strong women who are going through the same thing as you. Check online, find local support groups for menopausal women, or ask your doctor for information on community groups you could join. You could even look on social media and find Facebook support groups that suit your needs.

Fear of the unknown, not understanding what is happening to you, or feeling like no-one else is going through the same thing can usually worsen low mood and anxiety. Surround yourself with other women who are in the same situation can help you feel stronger, more confident, and ultimately, more positive within yourself.

## Seek Help if You Need It

The self-help methods that I mentioned will help you to feel more upbeat and help you be more in control of your mood and any anxiety you may experience. However, there is a fine line between feeling low and being depressed. It is vital to recognise this as struggling with low mood for too long can lead to depression.

For many people, admitting they are feeling depressed, anxious, agitated, etc. can be a huge uphill battle, but you must take that first step. Visit your doctor and be open about how you are feeling. You do not have to struggle and there are many treatment options your doctor may be able to explore with you in order to find the one that suits you best. Seeing a counsellor and receiving help with your feelings is worth considering. Or HRT could be the right option for you. It can help with mood-related menopausal symptoms. But there are also other options available that you can explore with your doctor.

Simply know that help is there if you need it, and you do not have to struggle your way through the menopause feeling less than yourself. Mental health is something we all need to learn to take just as seriously as our physical health.

## Key Points

- The menopause can cause mood swings, agitation, stress, anxiety and low confidence.

- Problems with mental health as a result of the menopause should not be ignored, and you should seek help from your doctor if you find these symptoms particularly troublesome.

- You can use several self-help methods to boost your mood, including exercising regularly, changing your diet, trying mindfulness with yoga, and others.

- HRT may be offered to you if you are struggling with mood during the menopause, but this is not something you have to take if you do not want to. I suggest that you talk to your doctor about alternatives.

- Remember to seek support from family, friends, and other women who are also going through the same thing as you.

- Always reach out for help if you are struggling with your mental health.

# Chapter 6

## Where Has Your Desire Gone?

With hormones causing all manner of confusion and upset within your body during the perimenopause and menopause, it is hardly surprising that sex is likely to be the last thing on your mind.

During the menopause, many women experience decreased desire, however it is equally as possible that your libido will shoot through the roof and your experience will be very different. Again, you have hormones to thank for all of this, but understanding how you can deal with a loss of libido in particular is a vital part of overcoming the struggles of the menopause.

You might think that lacking sex drive is not a big deal in the grand scheme of things, and for some women it probably is not, but if your partner's needs and expectations are different, then it can be quite difficult for both of you to deal with it. As a result, you might experience problems within your relationship and start noticing that your confidence drops. Many women feel more confident when they are having regular sex with their partner, and losing the desire for it or experiencing vaginal dryness, can drastically affect the way they feel about themselves.

There are several difficulties with the loss of libido. Firstly, some women can be very sexually active, but they begin to notice changes occurring in this department when they approach the menopause. You might start to feel confused as to why you are not feeling the desire as much anymore, or in some cases not at all. This could take your confidence away or even make you feel unattractive.

Secondly, you might start experiencing relationship issues because of this. Your partner needs to understand very clearly why you are feeling this way, which requires you to have open and honest communication with each other. Otherwise, your partner might conclude that you are not sexually attracted to them anymore. In some cases, that can cause serious issues within a relationship.

I believe that sexual intimacy between couples is important for maintaining a connection and keeping the desire alive, and if you fail to talk to your partner and let them know what is going on, it could be damaging for your relationship. Therefore, it is crucial that you open up and perhaps let your partner help you too; your partner may turn out to be your main ally against the menopause if you share your problems with them.

Of course, we have already explored the fact that hormonal imbalances cause your loss of libido, with dwindling testosterone levels being the main culprit. If you want to, you can take testosterone supplements, but these do come with their fair share of side effects, which may not be very beneficial when you weigh up the pros versus the cons. If you want to explore this possibility, consulting your doctor might be a good idea, and make sure to listen to both sides of the argument before making a final decision.

# Why is Libido Affected During the Menopause?

For some women, being menopausal simply means having no interest in sex. We know about the hormonal side of things, but what else can cause loss of libido during the menopause? It is not all about oestrogen, progesterone and testosterone for once. There are also a few other issues leading to these menopausal symptoms.

I have already mentioned the fact that during the menopause many women put on weight and find it harder to lose. Any excess weight can change the way you feel about yourself and affect your body confidence. Feeling this way might prevent you from being intimate with your partner and also stop you from enjoying sex.

Another common reason for the loss of libido with menopausal women is caused by the symptoms which they experience. Menopausal symptoms can make you feel generally uncomfortable, e.g. hot flushes, night sweats, and feeling tired in general. These can drastically reduce your desire to have sex.

Another symptom that is sex-related is vaginal dryness. These two symptoms are often interlinked and can cause upheaval in your relationship, and can drastically affect your confidence, if you allow them to.

Other reasons, such as feeling low in mood, anxious, or depressed, will undoubtedly affect your sexual desire. Suffering from depression can cause a lack of interest in sex, and it is usually one of the first symptoms that people notice. It is not surprising that women going through the menopause will not feel like having sex when their mood is affected.

Sex is supposed to be enjoyable, something that brings you closer to your partner. Therefore, it is understandable why both parties might feel unhappy with the situation you find yourself in, and frustrated about the issues you are experiencing.

If your lack of libido prevents you from enjoying this part of your relationship with your partner, it is important not to feel guilty about how this affects both of your lives. Both you and your partner must understand that this is not something you are choosing not to do, therefore communicating with each other during this time is vital.

Showing understanding towards each other's needs will strengthen your relationship and help you explore how to be intimate and close in other ways. Communicating your worries with your partner and respecting each other's wishes is vital at any stage of your relationship.

# Can You Boost Your Libido?

As I have already mentioned, a reduced sex drive can create problems in the relationship and talking to your partner about it is important. Being honest about how you are feeling can help you explore your relationship intimacy and find different ways to be close to each other. However, we will cover relationship issues later in this chapter.

There are some ways you can try and boost your libido, and get yourself in the mood if you do miss a little heat.

### Discuss HRT or Testosterone with Your Doctor

HRT might be able to help you with low libido and it could be an option for you if you choose to take it. As discussed previously, it can help with other menopausal symptoms too.

Throughout your life, your testosterone levels gradually decline and this can have a tremendous effect on your sex drive. There are also other benefits of testosterone such as maintaining muscle and bone strength and having normal cognitive functioning. If HRT is not helping you, then taking testosterone supplements could be another option for you. The issue with testosterone, however, is that it can, in some cases, cause excessive hair growth and acne for some women. It is important to be aware of this side effect before you decide to take it.

### Try Lubricants

Some women use lubricants to make the whole process easier. This ensures sex is more comfortable and enjoyable. Many couples choose to use lubricants as part of their sex life regardless, so definitely give it a try.

### Regular Exercise

Exercise is recommended for every menopausal side effect. It is an almost magical solution! Regular exercise releases those feel-good endorphins which can trigger sexual arousal and boost circulation which is useful for women who are trying to feel more in the mood.

Exercising will make you feel better in yourself and that could be enough to enhance your desire.

### *Try Kegel Exercises*

Kegel exercises are commonly used to strengthen the pelvic floor, especially during aging and after pregnancy, but it can be used for other reasons too. When you regularly do Kegel exercises you are boosting the circulation, which can make sex more enjoyable.

If you have never done Kegel exercises before, try this:

- First, you need to find the pelvic floor muscles to contract in the first place. When you urinate, you would contract your pelvic floor to stop the stream. That is the muscle you are looking for.

- Once you have figured out the right muscle, squeeze it for five seconds, counting slowly and steadily.

- Release the squeeze as you slowly and steadily count to five again.

- The ideal amount of exercises to do is 10 repetitions and you should try and do them three times per day. You might have to build up slowly, but that should be your aim.

Regularly practising Kegel exercises will help the blood flow, lubrication and sensitivity of the vagina which will make sex much more enjoyable.

### Cognitive Behavioural Therapy (CBT)

A possible treatment method for women who feel distressed from their low libido is to try CBT. It is a form of mindset training therapy used for a wide range of different problems and conditions. It can help you deal with the menopause symptoms that relate to your mood, and if your libido is affected directly because of that, you might find this therapy very helpful.

During the menopause and especially during the postmenopausal period it is very common to experience vaginal dryness. It causes discomfort and can make intercourse extremely uncomfortable and even painful. When you combine the possibility of vaginal dryness with the chance of a reduced libido, you can see why menopausal women are struggling with the idea of sex during this time of life. Sex is supposed to be fun, intimate and carefree — yet many women struggle with pain and discomfort.

In the next section, we will explore why vaginal dryness can be a problem for women, debunk your worries about whether it is dangerous or not, and figure out how to manage the problem overall.

## How to Overcome Vaginal Dryness

You have learnt so far that low levels of oestrogen and progesterone are responsible for most of the problems that occur during the menopause, and it is certainly the cause for vaginal dryness.

Some women only notice vaginal dryness as a problem during sexual intercourse, but others notice it more regularly. It can even happen while walking or wearing tight clothes. This is a massive problem for some postmenopausal women when oestrogen and progesterone are at an all-time low. As a result, the vagina is dry, and there is a risk of developing a condition called atrophic vaginitis or atrophy.

The medical name does sound scary, but it is a very common condition that affects many women; some women have this and are not even aware of it. Atrophic vaginitis or vaginal atrophy is when the vagina's tissues are not being nourished by oestrogen and progesterone, and as a result, they can become thinner. Simply wearing tight underwear can cause irritation and pain, sometimes resulting in bleeding. Of course, any bleeding after the menopause should be investigated by your doctor, and irritated vaginal atrophy or vaginitis can often be the cause of it.

Vaginal dryness is not dangerous per se, and the conditions associated with it will not cause you any real harm, but it is an uncomfortable and sometimes extremely painful condition to have. Thankfully it is possible to sort it out quite easily, and it is something we will explore next. I will give you some suggestions on what you can do to resolve it, so that your quality of life is not affected by this problem.

- *Have sex* – Regular sex has been shown to keep vaginal tissues healthy and help to reduce vaginal dryness and the possibility of atrophy after the menopause. It is quite ironic that loss of libido is one of the main symptoms of the menopause and even after the menopause, and as a result you might not feel like helping yourself to one of the best routes towards less vaginal dryness.

- *Use vaginal moisturisers regularly* – Using vaginal moisturisers every few days can reduce vaginal dryness and defend against the possibility of atrophy. Look for brands such as KY Jelly or Replens.

- *Use lubricants during sex* – Applying a few drops of lubricant just before sex can help to make the whole thing more comfortable and therefore more enjoyable for you and your partner. This will also help reduce pain and, as a result, you are more likely to relax and not always anticipate a painful reaction. Women who experience a large degree of vaginal dryness can lead to another potential problem called dyspareunia. It is persistent pain which usually occurs during sex, but can also happen before and after. In some cases, this can be very painful and can ruin a woman's sex life, but treatment is about learning to relax and allowing the vaginal muscles to do the same. Sexual responses are just as psychological as they are physiological, so be sure to focus on relaxation and take your time, if this is a problem for you.

- *Vaginal oestrogen* – Your doctor may prescribe you vaginal oestrogen at a low dose, which you can apply either as a cream, take as a tablet, or insert in a ring form. This approach helps to nourish the vaginal tissues and puts back some of the oestrogen you lack, due to the menopause. This will help to avoid vaginal atrophy and reduce the problem. However, vaginal oestrogen is not for everyone and if you have had breast cancer in the past or have a strong family history of it, you will need to discuss this carefully with your doctor to weigh up the pros and cons versus the risks.

- *Vaginal suppository (dehydroepiandrosterone)* – Your doctor might suggest a vaginal suppository that you insert every night, containing DHEA or dehydroepiandrosterone. This can help if you are suffering from painful intercourse as a result of vaginal dryness. A suppository such as this will help to nourish the tissues and help you relax as a result.

- *Ospemifene tablets* – This medication helps with painful intercourse caused by vaginal atrophy and dryness, but if you or anyone in your family has had breast cancer, this solution is not suitable for you.

In conclusion, I just want to say that if you are suffering from vagina dryness and it is affecting your life, you do not have to face it without help; it is simply a case of finding the right route forwards for your situation. There are many ways you can help to nourish your vaginal area and make everything less painful and more comfortable, whether you are attempting to have sex or not.

If this is a big problem for you, be sure to speak to your doctor as there are some prescription treatments you can try for severe cases. This is especially relevant if you notice dryness and discomfort during the day, when walking, sitting, or when wearing particular types of clothes.

## Talk to Your Partner

If you are in a relationship, it is vital that you are open and honest about your feelings with your partner and that you have honest communication with each other. Your partner may not understand the symptoms of the menopause and what is happening inside your body. Therefore, communicating your issues, worries, and desires is the key.

Whilst you should certainly never feel guilty for your libido problem, you also need to understand how the situation can impact upon your partner. Being honest and communicating openly is vital. It would be best if you talked to your partner to get them to understand and be sympathetic towards your situation.

By becoming emotionally closer to your partner in this way, you might also notice that your libido starts to come back a little. There are other ways to be intimate with your partner without having sexual intercourse, so spend time together, make date nights a priority, go back to holding hands, kissing, and caressing each other, and these forms of intimacy might help to boost your libido. If nothing else, they will bring you closer together as a couple and that could give you the extra boost of support you need to overcome the challenges you are facing in the menopause.

In some cases, sex drive can be a little like a muscle you work out at the gym. The more you work on it, the stronger it becomes. So, if your lack of or lower libido is a problem for you, work on making it stronger via non-sexual intimacy and see if it starts to trickle back into your life slowly. Many women find that it does.

However, after all this discussion about low libido, perhaps you are one of the women who notice a higher sex drive during the menopause! In that case, it could be a good thing or a bad thing for you; however, your partner is likely to find it a fantastic new development!

## Key Points

- Loss of libido is very common during the menopause and can also be connected to weight gain, loss of confidence or low mood.

- You must communicate with your partner to ensure that relationship problems do not occur due to a lack of sexual intimacy.

- There are a few ways to increase libido, including considering HRT or testosterone treatment, lubricants, CBT and regular exercise.

- Vaginal dryness is a common side effect of the menopause caused by reduced sex hormones, and it can contribute to loss of libido due to uncomfortable intercourse.

- Using vaginal moisturisers and lubricants are the most common ways to overcome vaginal dryness.

- Work on becoming emotionally closer to your partner during this time to maintain or even to improve your relationship.

# Chapter 7

# The Importance of Avoiding Toxins

As if we do not have enough to deal with during the menopause, it is important to be aware of outside influences that may cause more problems.

In this case, I am talking about toxins in general healthcare products.

Did you know that anything from shampoo to body lotion, and makeup remover to moisturiser can contain chemicals which can play havoc with your hormones? Also, pesticides and other harmful substances are used during the manufacturing process of certain fresh produce, which can also affect your hormones.

During the menopause you have enough going on, there is plenty to throw your hormonal balance out of sync as it is, so being aware of the toxins that can add to your troubles is vital. You can then work to decrease them and possibly even reduce your symptoms considerably.

In this chapter, we will look at why some toxins can affect your hormones, the ones you should try and avoid, and how you can find alternatives, so you are not missing out on any of your favourite health and beauty products.

## Why Are Toxins Troublesome During the Menopause?

Certain products contain chemical-based ingredients to prolong their shelf life, add attractive colours to their appearance, or boost the effectiveness of a natural ingredient. On the whole, many of these ingredients are considered "safe", although only in small amounts. What that "safe" label does not take into account is the effect that the ongoing use can have on the body and how it affects your endocrine system.

We already know that the endocrine system is responsible for many of your body's hormones. This can affect the big three hormones, which are affected during the menopause too — oestrogen, progesterone, and testosterone. By using products with a high amount of chemicals or toxins, you are certainly adding fuel to the fire.

Your hormones are already out of balance naturally at this stage of your life, but by continuing to use products that include toxins, you are increasing the detrimental effects, and therefore worsening your menopausal symptoms. The worst aspect of it all is that many women have no idea that their health and beauty products may have this effect on their symptoms, and they continue using them without even realising the dangers.

Some of the most common toxins which you need to avoid are parabens, ureas and sulphate. In the next section I will give you a comprehensive list, but you have no doubt heard of at least two of them.

Whilst the health and beauty industry has made a concerted effort to reduce the amount of toxins in their products, simply because the ingredients list of products are now subject to more scrutiny than ever before, they are still in there albeit in smaller amounts. By cutting these harmful chemicals out completely, you could help to reduce your hot flushes, night sweats, and other troublesome symptoms, simply by changing your beauty routine a little.

These toxins are known as "endocrine disrupting chemicals", and this means that they cause your hormones to be completely deranged. That is not what you need right now!

Your body cannot tell the difference between many of these toxins (which mimic the effects of oestrogen) and natural oestrogen, which can cause extra stress within your body and increase the number of menopausal symptoms you are experiencing, linked to your hormones. Besides, they can damage your insulin-producing cells, disrupt the hormones released from your thyroid gland, and cause your body's natural detoxing system to be completely out of sync.

Hormones are very closely linked. It is common for women to gain weight during the menopause because the distortion in oestrogen and progesterone also affects ghrelin and leptin, which tells you when you are full or hungry.

I have already mentioned the fact that thyroid hormones can be disrupted due to the imbalance of oestrogen. All hormones affect one another in some way, so when toxins affect one hormone, you can expect a knock-on effect with the others, particularly when it comes to oestrogen imbalance.

## Hidden Toxins in Personal Care Products

Most health and beauty products are applied to the skin and absorbed. If products contain these toxins, or fake/synthetic oestrogen (more on that shortly), they are absorbed into the blood stream and cause your existing imbalance to deteriorate.

Let's look at some of the most common toxins you need to try and cut out of your health and beauty routine. You can learn what is in each of your favourite products by simply reading the ingredients on the back — manufacturers now have to mention if they include any of these toxins, so it is worthwhile becoming better informed about the contents of the products you use.

- **BPA** – This is a chemical which is regularly used in plastic products, but it is used in some health and beauty products, packaged to actually imitate oestrogen, thereby acting as a synthetic, or fake, oestrogen. BPAs have links with various types of cancer, reproductive issues, heart disease, and early cases of puberty.

- **Dioxin** – Dioxin is used in many different products and packaging types. Dioxin is famous for disrupting sex hormones and can stay in the body for quite a long time. It is also very hard to avoid, so you need to become alert and cautious when reading packaging before using products.

- **Atrazine** – Studies with atrazine have found that it interacts with sex hormones. Again, we are looking at a further disruption to oestrogen here. Atrazine also has a link with breast tumors and puberty delays, amongst many other general health issues.

- **Phthalates** – There are many studies which link phthalates to hormonal changes and problems with the thyroid gland. Phthalates also affect the male reproductive system but have been shown to cause havoc with hormones in general.

- **Parabens** – More and more health and beauty products are trying to cut out parabens in their products, but this is a work in progress for many. Parabens imitate oestrogen and is likely to cause your current menopausal symptoms to change or worsen, due to a further imbalance. Parabens have also been shown to cause problems with other hormones whilst also affecting the reproductive system.

- **Sulphates** – A little like parabens, sulphates can be found in many health and beauty products, although there is a concerted effort to try and reduce this. Sulphates act as synthetic oestrogen, thereby causing many menopausal symptoms to worsen, whilst also increasing the risk of disruption to thyroid hormones.

It is not only health and beauty products you need to be careful of. Many chemicals and toxins can be found in various foods, generally originating from how they are grown or manufactured. There is a concerted push to reduce manufacturing that includes fake hormones or pesticides, but they continue to occur.

If you can, I suggest that you shop organically. Yes, these products can cost a little more, but they are a much healthier alternative to conventionally grown produce. They contain a higher level of antioxidants and have far less synthetic chemicals.

Eating organic foods will help you avoid the likelihood of ingesting pesticides and other manufacturing toxins. Clean eating helps menopausal women to manage their symptoms better.

Buying a filter for your water is a wise investment. There are many contaminants found in drinking water and even though this is classed as safe to drink, it may contain traces of toxins that could affect your hormones. If you drink filtered water only, you will avoid this risk, and you will be drinking cleaner and healthier water as a result.

## Alternative Products to Try

First things first, not all health and beauty products contain toxins, and you should become used to reading labels and knowing what to look for. In addition to the toxins mentioned earlier, you should also avoid any product which lists the following ingredients on their packaging:

- Fragrance

- Artificial colours

- Petroleum

- Formaldehyde

- Preservatives

- Foaming agents

- Antibacterial agents

- Plasticisers

- Siloxanes

- PEG compounds

The best suggestion I can give you is to cut out some of the products which you know contain toxins and see how you feel after a week or two. If you notice a difference in your menopausal symptoms or you simply feel better in yourself, try and find an alternative to that particular product. It is not always easy to pinpoint one specific product, especially if you have a bathroom cabinet brimming with different lotions, potions, and creams! By swapping some of the products you use most often, perhaps one by one, you will be able to identify which is causing you the biggest issue.

Try looking for products that contain organic or natural ingredients only. These will be marked as such, but again, read the labels to be sure. You might also like to try making your own products in some cases, such as body scrubs, exfoliators, moisturisers, etc. You might not be able to do this with all your favourite health and beauty products, but if you check online you will find a range of "recipes" to make completely natural products. This can also be quite fun, and you could gift these to friends too.

Avoiding toxins can not only help you with your menopausal symptoms but can lead to better overall health and well-being and reduce risk factors for developing chronic or severe diseases.

## Key Points

This chapter has covered the importance of understanding how toxins and chemicals contained within health and beauty products may affect your hormones. You might not have even been aware of this before, but you may have heard about a few of the ingredients mentioned in this book.

By reducing your exposure to toxins, you may find that your menopausal symptoms reduce or even themselves out a little. Of course, this also reduces your risk of developing serious health problems as a result of too much exposure over time.

The main points to remember from this chapter are:

- Certain toxins found in health and beauty products can mimic the effects of oestrogen, as well as progesterone and testosterone. The body does not know how to differentiate between natural and synthetic oestrogen, therefore these products add to your menopausal problems.

- Manufacturers are now required to list all ingredients on their packaging, so in order to avoid your exposure to common toxins, always read labels thoroughly.

- Parabens, sulphates and BPA are three of the most common types of toxins that affect hormones, however, there is a long list of the most dangerous types to avoid.

- Look for products that are labelled as organic or natural.

- Shop for organic produce to avoid your exposure to dangerous pesticides, and other toxins used in the manufacturing process.

- Use a water filter to cut out any contaminants in your water.

- Try cutting out products one by one and seeing how you feel in yourself; this will show you if one particular product and its associated toxins are affecting your hormones or not.

# Chapter 8

# Palpitations and Headaches, What is The Deal?

The menopause can throw some very odd symptoms at you and two of the most difficult to deal are palpitations and headaches. They occur in two very different parts of the body, but they can be related or unrelated, and can be part of your menopausal journey.

Why does the menopause cause these particular symptoms?

In the earlier chapters, I blamed hormones for almost everything that happens to us, and they definitely cause these occasional headaches and palpitations.

The reason for this is because of the changing levels of hormones in your body. It is common for palpitations to occur during hot flushes as you notice your heart beating a little faster. And for women who experience hormone-related headaches that often occur during or before their monthly cycle, they could start having severe and frequent headaches.

Palpitations usually disappear as quickly as they appear, but they can be upsetting whilst they are there. If you notice you are suffering from palpitations, sit down, breathe steadily and wait for it to pass. It is important to remain calm and remember that nothing is going to hurt you; most of the time palpitations are harmless.

In this chapter, I am going to focus on these two troubling symptoms and give you some advice on how to reduce them.

Some women may go through the menopause and never notice even one palpitation, whilst some may have lots of them. Some women may go through the menopause and not have more headaches than they usually would have. Some women have them regularly. It is a personalised deal and it is important to know what your version of normal is.

## The Importance of Monitoring Palpitations and Headaches

Whilst both palpitations and headaches are not harmful in general, they can occur due to underlying causes in some situations. That means it is vital that you monitor them and get anything checked out that does not feel right to you. This advice is the same for all other symptoms I have mentioned in this book.

If you notice that you are getting more headaches and palpitations, it is good to keep a symptom diary. This will give your doctor more information to work with, and they will be able to understand whether there is a pattern to your symptoms. This will help your doctor to diagnose your problem more easily.

In rare cases, both palpitations and headaches can be due to more sinister reasons, but these are few and far between, and both symptoms are very common in regular life. In fact, both can be caused by stress, which we are going to cover in more detail next.

# The Link with Stress and How to Reduce It

Stress can cause all manner of symptoms to occur within the body and most of the time you do not even know you are stressed!

We live in stressful times and that means that most of us are operating within a constantly heightened state of awareness. The body has its own stress response, more commonly known as the "fight or flight" response.

When your brain observes something and thinks of it as a threat, it gives your body everything it needs to either fight the danger, or run away from it. The problem is that your brain will always remember negative past experiences and perceive new situations as a threat. This might make you feel constantly stressed out and result in increased cortisol levels. Cortisol is the stress hormone, contributing to the imbalance of hormones you already have due to the menopause.

Stress can cause headaches and it can also cause heart palpitations. When stress is prolonged, the body does not know how to differentiate between a normal state and a stressed state. As a result, regular uncomfortable symptoms occur, such as trouble sleeping, appetite problems (eating too little or too much), low mood, agitation and headaches.

The good news is that you have more control than you realise. Stress might seem like it is controlling your life, but you can change your lifestyle and take back control of your own ship.

It might take a little time, but little by little you will notice that you feel better in yourself. There are no downsides to focusing on stress reduction, so make this your aim whether you are suffering from palpitations and headaches or not.

In today's society, we are constantly subjected to stress. It is such a chronic state of being, that we might not even be aware of all the ways in which we might be experiencing stress. In order to manage your stress effectively it is important to find out what is causing it. Identifying your stressors is the first step towards having a stress-free life.

The following exercise can help you to recognise your stressors and find different ways of removing them from your life. Follow these five simple steps:

1. Take a piece of paper or a notebook and brainstorm your stressors – It might be something that is massive, or it might be very small. If it is affecting your stress levels, it is important. Never pass something off as too small; if it is bothering you, it is large enough to take notice of.

2. Write them down.

3. Is there one thing you can pinpoint, or are there several?

4. Work out how you can address those problems. Remember, some of them you may not be able to address immediately.

5. Draw a plan to overcome your stressors. Use the piece of paper or write it in your notebook. Working out a plan puts you in charge and creates a feeling of being in control of your life. It is a great confidence boost and an excellent motivational tool.

I hope that this exercise will help you to identify your stressors, so you can make changes that will help you reduce your stress levels.

Sitting down and doing some soul searching might not be enough for some people. If this is the case, I suggest you follow the rules for stress management. Most common tips include:

- Exercise regularly

- Reduce your caffeine and alcohol intake

- Reduce how much sugar you eat

- Do your best to get a good night's sleep

- Meditate and practice mindfulness

- Be positive

Stress is not something you should be inviting into your life, and learning how to reduce the amount of stress you are experiencing is vital for your health and happiness too. Of course, this will also help to reduce any troubling symptoms you are experiencing, including previously mentioned headaches and palpitations.

Anxiety is another symptom of the menopause and it has a strong link with stress. It has been shown that stress aggravates the symptoms of anxiety. Therefore, you must learn the cause of your anxiety and understand its connection with stress. Some people feel shaky or distant when their anxiety is spiking, whilst others feel heavy and hot. Learn to recognise your feelings of anxiety, as this will help you to intervene if things start to deteriorate. Getting familiar with your triggers will help you to manage them better and reduce the severity they might have on your life. Many women learn to do this before the menopause, such is the prevalence of anxiety in modern society.

The constant attack of stress can lead to hormonal disorders like adrenal fatigue, in which your adrenal glands (responsible for producing your stress hormones) become overworked and begin to wear out. This leads to physical fatigue, lack of motivation and depression.

Metabolic disorders are hormonal as well, and conditions like insulin or leptin resistance can cause an increase in your stress hormones, which create a downward spiral of hormonal dysfunction.

Hormonal health is particularly fragile in menopausal women as their bodies naturally start to alter the production of hormones. This is perfectly normal and natural, but it does cause a shift in the entire endocrine system. By introducing outside factors to the mix, like diet and environment, this change then becomes exponentially more difficult for the body to adjust to.

# Natural Methods to Reduce Palpitations and Headaches

Palpitations and headaches might not be the worst of your menopausal problems. Perhaps you suffer from hot flushes far more than headaches, and maybe you do not have palpitations at all. However, you might be plagued with them. In either situation, knowing what to do to reduce them naturally is a good thing.

I am aware that today many people reach for painkillers even when they feel the slightest pain somewhere in the body. I understand that sometimes it is necessary to take them in order to numb the pain, but I am not a fan of taking them regularly.

There are countless reasons why you might be experiencing heart palpitations or headaches. It could be because of some underlying condition that you have, or changes in your hormone levels, or due to stress.

Here, I would like to highlight natural processes to deal with the issues of palpitations and headaches.

### *Natural Methods to Reduce Palpitations:*

- **Regularly use relaxation techniques** – Deep breathing, exercise, and meditation are ideal ways to relax your mind and body and reduce palpitations. When you are experiencing a palpitation, try to focus on your breathing and slow it down. As a result, the palpitation will pass much faster and you will not become anxious or worried about the feeling. Remember, palpitations can last for a few seconds or a few minutes, but they are not dangerous, so do not be too worried about them. You should also try practising relaxation in general, as this will help you get a good night's sleep, something that can be difficult for some menopausal women to achieve.

- *Cut down on stimulants* – Try to do your best to cut down on stimulants. Consuming stimulants such as caffeine, tobacco, alcohol and sugar are bad habits that could be extremely damaging to your health, and are also known to increase the risk of palpitations. Remember that caffeine can also be in other drinks aside from coffee, such as cola, tea, and even in chocolate. If you can cut down on the amount of sugar you consume, that will positively affect your hot flushes and the number of palpitations you have.

- *Work on your vagus nerve* – The vagus nerve carries signals between your brain and throughout the rest of your body. By stimulating your vagus nerve, you can learn to reduce the number of palpitations you experience as you can slow down your heart rate to a steady and regular rhythm. This may not mean that palpitations are never experienced, but they should be far less frequent. A few ways to do this include:

- o Exposure to cold temperatures (do this with caution, however, as too much cold too quickly can cause shock – a cold compress is enough)

- o Breathing deeply and slowly

- o Humming and singing

- o Meditating

- o Eating omega-3 fatty acids (found in fish)

- o Consuming probiotics (try yogurt, traditional buttermilk, kefir, sauerkraut and other fermented foods)

- o Exercise

- o Try massage

These are all healthy things to work on regardless of your aim, but by stimulating the vagus nerve, you may be able to reap the benefits of reducing the amount of palpitations.

- • ***Reduce your salt intake*** – Too much salt is not good for your health and may contribute to your palpitations. Make sure that you cut down on the amount of salt you consume throughout the day and be wary of added salt in packaged or processed foods. Eating a healthy diet overall can help reduce your menopausal symptoms and improve your health and general well-being.

- **Drink plenty of water** – Water is the magical elixir of life in so many ways. Make sure that you drink enough water every single day, without fail. There is some debate over how much is enough, but the general consensus is that eight glasses a day is sufficient. If you struggle with the bland taste, add a squeeze of fresh lemon and lime to jazz it up.

- **Exercise regularly** – Exercise is vital on so many levels. It helps to keep your heart healthy, regulates stress levels, reduces anxiety, and as a result, can help to reduce the number of palpitations you have, or even remove them completely. I suggest that you find a type of exercise that you enjoy and start doing it just a few hours per week. This is enough to keep you in better shape and the results will filter down through the rest of your body.

*Natural Methods to Reduce Headaches:*

- **Drink plenty of water** – Being dehydrated can cause a headache, so it might not even be your hormonal imbalance that is causing the pain, but the fact that you are dehydrated. Before reaching for a painkiller, sit down, relax and drink a glass of water. See how you feel after a short while. However, drinking plenty of water throughout the day, every day, will reduce the number of headaches you experience in general, whilst helping you to have more energy and even regulate your appetite.

- *Increase your magnesium intake* – You can take a magnesium supplement if you choose to, but you can go down the natural route and try getting your daily magnesium amount from your diet. Foods rich in magnesium include avocados, nuts, legumes, tofu, whole grains, seeds, and fatty fish types. You can also find magnesium in dark chocolate, but remember that moderation is vital as chocolate can also cause headaches in some people. If you feel like a supplement might be a better route for you, speak to your doctor before you begin, especially if you are currently taking any other medications or you have any pre-existing medical conditions. The green light from your doctor will give you peace of mind.

- *Cut down on alcohol intake* – Alcohol dehydrates your body, which is always going to lead to a headache. A hangover the next morning is partly down to dehydration, so remember to reduce your alcohol intake and see if your headaches decrease. This does not mean that you cannot enjoy the odd glass of wine, but it does mean that everything in moderation is the key. Alcohol is also a stimulant, so do not be tempted to drink an alcoholic drink before bed in the hope that it will help you sleep — it might help you nod off quicker but you will wake up during the night as the effects wear off, and you will probably need to get up and use the toilet more often, which is going to disrupt your sleep.

- *Make sure you get enough sleep* – Poor sleep is always going to lead to a headache and when you are not rested, a whole host of other problems come your way. Certainly, an insufficient amount of sleep and poor sleep quality are the main issues for menopausal women, but doing your best to try and get a regular seven to eight hours of sleep every night is important. Make sure that you go to bed and wake up at the same time every day, avoid stimulants (coffee, tea, smoking, alcohol) in the hours before bed, and lay off your phone usage an hour or so before you plan to sleep. Your sleeping environment needs to be comfortable ensuring that you are not too hot or too cold. Making an effort to improve your sleeping pattern is extremely important. Lack of sleep leads to sleep deprivation in the long-term and it must not be ignored. It does not just cause headaches, but can cause a myriad of other health issues too.

- *Avoid foods which have a high histamine amount* – Some women experience migraines or severe headaches when they eat a diet high in histamine. Histamine is a compound found within the body which cells release whenever you become ill or get injured. It is part of the immune system and encourages the inflammatory response. Histamine stimulates the dilation of capillaries within the body, which could lead to headaches. Cutting out foods high in histamine could therefore reduce your headaches naturally. Avoid fermented drinks, including alcohol (beer is the worst for this), fermented foods (including yogurt), avocados, dried varieties of fruit, eggplant, shellfish, smoked meat, processed meats, and spinach. You might look at that list and wonder why super-foods such as avocados and fermented foods, which are high in probiotics are there. It is because some women do not respond too well to these foods, therefore it is always a good idea to work out whether you fall into this bracket by cutting them out gradually one by one, and paying attention to how your body will respond to this change.

- *Use a cold compress* – Whilst you are suffering from a headache, try a cold compress across your head, with a glass of water on the side. Sit down with your head back and relax or lay down if you prefer. Close your eyes and focus on your breathing. You may find that after a short while the headache reduces without the need to take a painkiller. Make sure that the compress is not too cold, as this could cause the headache to worsen; cool is the aim here, not freezing.

- **_Try essential oils_** – Aromatherapy has been around for centuries, and the use of essential oils means that you can try and reduce many ailments without medical means; one of those ailments is headaches. Lavender oil, rosemary oil, peppermint oil, chamomile oil and eucalyptus oil are all recommended for reducing headaches and inflammation whilst lavender is also great for promoting sleep. You can add this to your bath water, place it on your wrists, spray a little onto your pillow, or simply inhale it via a diffuser.

- **_B complex vitamins_** – Some women find that taking a B complex vitamin supplement can help reduce the number of headaches they get, particularly migraines. If headaches are causing the issue for you, you can talk to your doctor about possibly adding this supplement to your routine. Alternatively, you can go down the natural route and add foods into your diet which are naturally high in this vitamin. These include salmon, liver, organ meats, eggs, leafy greens, milk, mussels, oysters, clams, beef, and legumes.

A few of the methods for reducing headaches are also useful for reducing the frequency of palpitations, and vice versa. However, the good news is that they are all quite easy to incorporate into your daily routine, and they will all give you other health benefits too.

## Key Points

In this chapter, I have shared in-depth information about palpitations and headaches during the menopause. Again, not all women will find these symptoms to be a problem, but if they are troublesome for you, you can see that there are many natural ways to reduce them.

As with all the symptoms we have covered so far, headaches and palpitations during the menopause are mostly down to the hormonal fluctuations and imbalances you are experiencing during the perimenopause and the menopause phase. These can also continue after the menopause, for a few years into the postmenopausal period. If you are at all worried, you should go and see your doctor and get checked.

Whilst both of these symptoms are very common during the menopausal period, they are sometimes a sign of something a little more serious. Ruling that out will give you peace of mind, and from there you can work towards reducing these symptoms via natural means.

The main points to remember from this chapter are:

- Headaches and palpitations are common symptoms during the menopause.

- Not all women experience these symptoms, but many do. You could experience both symptoms together or separately, and one may be more severe than another.

- Palpations are rarely serious, but if you are worried, you should get them checked, as they could be a sign of a heart issue.

- Similarly, headaches are rarely severe, but they can be linked to other conditions, so if you are worried, get these checked with your doctor.

- Fluctuating hormone levels are the cause of both of these symptoms during this time of life.

- Stress can have a powerful effect on both palpitations and headaches, so naturally reducing stress is a good starting point.

- Both headaches and palpitations can be reduced via natural methods. Try to get enough sleep, drink plenty of water, and minimise exposure to stimulants.

# Chapter 9

# The Link With Osteoporosis

One of the main words that is associated with the menopause is "osteoporosis".

It may sound frightening, but when you dig a little deeper and understand more about it, you will realise that there are many things you can do to reduce your risk of developing osteoporosis in later life. It is also very unlikely that every menopausal woman is going to develop osteoporosis, but falling oestrogen levels do put you at a higher risk than at other times in your life. Women are also more at risk than men.

However, before we get into the finer details of how to minimise your risk, we need to delve a little deeper into what osteoporosis is.

## What is Osteoporosis?

Osteoporosis is a long-term health problem that occurs as you age. Over time, bones weaken, and this makes them more likely to fracture and break more easily, than at any other time in your life. The role of oestrogen helps to keep the bones strong and flexible, and the problem arises during the menopause when women start experiencing falling levels of oestrogen, which contributes to the risks of developing osteoporosis.

There is no routinely performed test to find out whether you are at risk of developing osteoporosis. It is usually diagnosed when someone breaks a bone, and a bone density test is done that shows whether or not you have osteoporosis. This is not routinely done beforehand, unless there is a medical indicator for it, in which case the doctor may send you for a DEXA scan. This measures the density of your bones and gives an indication of what is going on.

Osteoporosis affects all bones, but there are some more common ones — wrist, hips and vertebrae, also known as your spinal bones. We quite frequently hear about older people having hip replacements due to fractures and weakening. This can often be because of osteoporosis.

As with any medical condition, osteoporosis can be mild, moderate, or severe. In the worst cases, even a sneeze or a heavy cough can lead to a broken rib or having a problem with a spinal bone.

As osteoporosis sets in, your posture can change. You might have seen some elderly people in the forward bending position. This is due to osteoporosis, as the bones in the spine become weak and brittle, and therefore cannot support the body as well as they did before.

When osteoporosis is diagnosed, it can be treated with medicines that strengthen the bones, but the medication will not always work. This is why it is always best to look at prevention rather than attempting to cure what has been damaged. There is no actual cure for osteoporosis either, so a healthy lifestyle is one of the best ways to prevent this condition.

It sounds like a rather grim outlook, but it is important to mention that not every menopausal woman is going to develop osteoporosis when she gets older. This also is not a problem that is going to affect you right now; you will not know whether this is a problem for you until you notice regularly broken bones, a few years or even decades into the future.

# How to Reduce Your Risk Factors for Osteoporosis

Whilst it is true that not every menopausal woman will develop osteoporosis in later life, it is something that you need to pay great attention to once you reach the postmenopausal stage. Osteoporosis can cause long-term pain when bones are weak and brittle, so you must do whatever you can right now to reduce this risk.

Both men and women can develop osteoporosis, but women are more likely to as a result of the loss of oestrogen during the menopause. This risk is further compounded if you undergo premature menopause or have had surgery to remove your ovaries.

So, what can you do to reduce the risk?

The good news is that there are steps you can start taking right now.

### Regular Exercise

Regular exercise is the best starting point. Aim for around two and a half hours every week, hitting a moderate level of intensity. This can be walking fast, cycling, jogging, or anything that gets you out of breath and pushes your heart rate up.

You should also add in some weight bearing and resistance exercises, as these are ideal for boosting bone density, helping you reduce your risk of developing osteoporosis. Strength and flexibility are what you need to aim for.

I suggest you do some muscle strengthening exercises two to three days a week, and make sure that you use all the main muscle groups.

My book *Get Fit and Healthy in Your Own Home in 20 Minutes or Less*, which is available on Amazon, is a fantastic resource for finding exercise routines to suit your needs. Inside the book, you will find plenty of exercises that cover warm-ups, stretching, and strength training for your upper and lower body. You will also find many simple and healthy ideas for breakfast, lunch, dinner, and snacks.

The ideas for weight-bearing exercises include jogging, dancing, skipping, climbing stairs, and jumping up and down. Remember to wear shoes that give proper support to your feet and ankles. If you are having back problems or you struggle with your knees, then I recommend swimming as it is a less intense exercise, but it still gives your muscles a great workout.

On the other hand, resistance exercises look a little different. These include using hand weights, doing press-ups or lunges, etc. If you have gym membership, you will find plenty of equipment there to help you perform this type of exercise. Otherwise, you can usually make use of household items, for example two cans of food work very well for hand weights. There are many ideas for different types of exercises in my book, which I mentioned earlier.

### Eat a Healthy Diet

So many of the menopausal symptoms we have looked at so far can be improved with eating healthily. A healthy diet is recommended as one of the main contributors to reducing the risks of osteoporosis.

Two main vitamins you need to help reduce your osteoporosis risk are calcium and vitamin D. Soon, I will talk about whether you can get these from a supplement, but first, let's explore natural methods.

Calcium helps to keep your bones healthy, as well as your teeth and nails. The recommended daily intake is 700mg per day and it is entirely possible to get that from your regular diet. Some of the foods which you can add to your daily diet include:

- Leafy greens (the darker, the better)

- Dried varieties of fruit

- Tofu

- Dairy products such as milk, cheese and yoghurt

Vitamin D works with calcium. It helps your body to absorb the calcium you are getting from food. Therefore, if you are deficient in vitamin D, the calcium you are consuming will not work efficiently.

Your daily intake of vitamin D needs to be 10 micrograms every day, and you can find vitamin D in the following foods:

- Red meat (it can increase your risk of heart disease when eaten in large quantities, therefore eat in moderation)

- Liver

- Oily varieties of fish such as herring, mackerel, sardines, and salmon

- Egg yolks

- Foods which are classified as "fortified", e.g. certain cereals — you will find this out by reading the packaging as it will be marketed as such

### Increase Your Vitamin D Intake via Sunlight

It is possible to boost your own natural vitamin D production by soaking up the sun. Of course, you need to practice sun safety, as sunburn and sunstroke are not attractive or healthy. I recommend you go out and enjoy benefits of the sun when it is not as intense but is wonderfully warm.

### Reduce Smoking and Drinking

Drinking alcohol and smoking can weaken bones over time and therefore contribute to your risk of developing osteoporosis. Smoking in particular has been shown to increase the likelihood of osteoporosis. As for drinking alcohol, it is recommended to stick to no more than 14 units per week to remain within healthy boundaries. Cutting down on drinking and stopping smoking can not only help you to prevent osteoporosis, but will also reduce many of your menopausal symptoms such as hot flushes.

## Should You Take Supplements?

It is possible to take supplements for both calcium and vitamin D to support your bone health, but it is always a good idea to speak to your doctor about it, and understand the side effects of any supplement you are thinking of taking. As I mentioned earlier, calcium can generally be consumed in a sufficient amount for your body via your diet, but you may find it a little harder to get enough vitamin D following that route.

As suggested already, you can soak up the sun and increase your vitamin D production levels, but there are no concrete guidelines on how long it takes to be in the sun to give you enough of it. With that in mind, you might want to consider taking a vitamin D supplement alongside a healthy diet packed with a variety of different vitamins and minerals.

## Key Points

In this chapter, you learnt how reduced oestrogen increases your risk of developing osteoporosis in later life. If you want to be happy and healthy in your later years, it is a good idea to start reducing your risk now.

Just because you are going through the menopause, it does not necessarily mean that you are going to develop osteoporosis, but it is a risk that you need to take seriously.

Here are the main points to remember from this chapter:

- Osteoporosis is the weakening of bones which typically happens in later life. It can occur as a result of low levels of oestrogen which contributes to your overall risk factor.

- Women who go through the menopause prematurely or who have had surgery to remove their ovaries have an increased risk.

- Osteoporosis varies in intensity and is indicated by the frequent breaking of bones, which can lead to long-term pain.

- Learning to reduce your risk of osteoporosis includes taking regular exercise, including moderate-level cardio, weight bearing and muscle strengthening exercises.

- Eating a healthy diet, packed with calcium and vitamin D, is important for strong and healthy bones.

- You can take a supplement of both vitamin D and calcium if you choose to.

- It is possible to boost your body's own vitamin D production by spending time in the sun.

# Conclusion

Every woman goes through the menopause. It is not something you can shy away from or prevent, but you can control it in terms of whether it is a happy and healthy experience or a very difficult one. The menopause does not just happen to you. It is something you can shape to a certain degree and learn how to handle via natural ways, and in some cases, with a little help from the medical world.

You can make numerous lifestyle changes to help with standard and troubling menopausal symptoms, or you can choose to take the medication in the form of HRT. Never feel that you are being forced to take HRT as this is something you decide for yourself. Your doctor may encourage this as a good route for reducing the menopause symptoms, but if you are still unsure whether it is the best option for you, you do not have to take it. There are many natural ways you can approach the issue and it is advisable to see how they work for you. Of course, you can always change your mind and ask for HRT again at a later stage if you are a suitable candidate for it.

The point is that you need to take control of your menopause and bend it to your will. It might sound impossible, but by reading this book you will hopefully have seen that it is entirely possible to do so. However, all of this requires a strong and positive mindset, with the determination to live a healthier and happier lifestyle.

A healthy and happy menopause is about focusing on your confidence and battling any troublesome symptoms. There is no "one size fits all" answer here, as every woman experiences a range of different symptoms, to varying degrees. What you can do, however, is read up on the most common and most troublesome symptoms and learn how to reduce their impact. The good news is that most of the advice for one troubling symptom will directly and positively impact many of the others. That means there is actually very little that you need to do, other than ensuring that your life in general is healthy and free of negative effects on your well-being.

Of course, that does not mean that you should just tolerate symptoms that are causing you problems. If you are struggling or you are worried about anything, you should speak to your doctor and seek reassurance and guidance. You may be going through the menopause for many years, and you might experience symptoms for up to 10 years — that is a lot of years to be dealing with symptoms that cause you discomfort or even distress. It is far better to speak to a health professional and find a way to reduce symptoms that trouble you, in a way that suits you. Thankfully, as you have learnt from this book, there are many options to choose from.

## Every Woman's Experience is Different

I would like you to remember that every woman has a slightly different experience when going through the menopause. You can compare notes with your friends, but just because one friend is having a terrible time with mood swings, it does not mean that you will have a bad time too. Similarly, you might be troubled by hot flushes and night sweats, but she might barely notice them. You might be experiencing anxiety, but your sister may never have problems with it. There is no way to predict the symptoms you are going to have and which ones will be worse for you and which will be less troublesome.

We are all different and that is what makes us so wonderful. Unique women can take on the world and that also means taking on the menopause and conquering it, one symptom at a time.

However, it is a good idea to seek support from women going through the same thing as you and communicate with your loved ones and let them know what is going on. You are not in this alone, and the more you cut yourself off and try to handle it alone, the harder it will be. Share your experience to the degree you feel comfortable with and remember to be kind to yourself during this time. You are experiencing a lot of changes in your body and these are bound to affect how you feel within yourself and about yourself.

Your menopausal experience does not have to be negative, and it does not have to be a stage in your life that you just "get through". It can be a time to realise your power, to understand your body, and to reclaim what is yours. You no longer have to deal with those troublesome monthly bleeds, no more PMT, and you can wave goodbye to pregnancy risk! Once the menopause is over, none of these things are a concern anymore and whilst you might still have symptoms for a few years afterwards, you can rest safe in the knowledge that they will not last forever. Whether that is a few months more or a few years more depends entirely on your body, but they will disappear in the end.

Hopefully you will have absorbed all the information in this book and understood what you need to do to make your menopausal journey easier.

I also hope that you learnt enough about health and well-being to pass that information onto your family members. Just because they are not going through the menopause, it does not mean they should not focus on health! When the entire household is eating healthily, it is far easier for you to do it too and stick to it. You will notice that with the support of your family, you will be able to get through your menopausal journey much more easily.

# Final Words

I want to say that we must not simply blame hormones for everything that happens to us. It is very easy to say "I'm fat because of my hormones", or "I'm stressed because of my hormones", or "I'm tired because of my hormones".

Yes, your hormones can affect your weight, mood and sleep, but paying attention to your diet, lifestyle and changing your attitude and behaviour towards the way you live your life, will significantly impact your hormones and your general well-being. Do not allow your hormones to control you. Make sure that you control YOU.

All that is left to do now is to wish you a healthy and happy menopause, full of empowerment, confidence, and the realisation that you are a truly unique and special woman who is not defined by the time of life she is going through.

Keep this book handy and refer to it whenever a new symptom comes your way, or whenever you want to change your approach to an existing one. Consider it your guide to achieving a happy, healthy, and perhaps even confidence-boosting menopause!

I wish you all the best!

Lots of love xx

Silvana

# Thank You

I hope you enjoyed this book!

Please consider leaving a review on Amazon – even if it is only a few sentences, it would be a huge help. Here is the link for your convenience. Go to http://viewbook.at/healthy-menopause. Your review will help other readers benefit from the information in this book.

Please visit bit.ly/silvana-signup to join the mailing list for updates on future books and to receive information about health, weight loss, and nutrition.

# About the Author

Silvana Siskov has spent more than 20 years working with people experiencing a variety of issues, such as mental health, eating disorders and weight management problems. Her speciality is giving sound advice with a strong focus on emotional support. She is also dedicated to helping clients find a strong direction in the areas of their lives where they need it the most.

Silvana helps establish clarity around the issues which her clients are facing in their everyday lives. This allows them to take control of their health and well-being and change their lifestyle towards the positive end of the scale. By doing this, they are able to achieve their own health goals and improve their confidence levels and develop a sense of self-worth.

Following some personal health issues, Silvana's interest in nutrition grew. This led her towards supporting clients on their weight loss journeys, giving them advice on nutrition and their dietary needs and helping them overcome pitfalls such as comfort eating.

From this experience, Get Your Sparkle Back: 10 Steps to Weight Loss and Overcoming Emotional Eating was born. The fantastic reaction to this book led her to write more, helping her clients to achieve their own lifestyle goals and feel more confident from within. The book *Live Healthy on a Tight Schedule* followed quickly, empowering readers to be far less dependent on external factors and to take more control of their lives. Shortly after this book was published, *Get Fit and Healthy in Your Own Home in 20 Minutes or Less* was written. This book continues to help Silvana's readers to work towards their health and weight loss goals.

The following two books that Silvana wrote were focused on the menopause. The first book in the series *Beat Your Menopause Weight Gain*, was very quickly followed by *Free Yourself From Hot Flushes and Night Sweats*. With these two books Silvana helps women to better manage their menopausal journey and to reduce symptoms brought by the menopause.

Silvana finds true pleasure in supporting her clients and working closely with them on a one-on-one basis. She also extends her work into the community, with talks and workshops for those who prefer a more sociable atmosphere.

Silvana's overall mission is to empower and motivate women, helping them to use their power from within and create a deeper connection to themselves. By doing so, they can achieve whatever they put their minds to, living their very best lives.

# Helpful Resources

*Books by Silvana Siskov:*

- *"Get Your Sparkle Back: 10 Steps to Weight Loss and Overcoming Emotional Eating."* The book is available on Amazon. Go to http://viewbook.at/sparkle.

- *"Live Healthy on a Tight Schedule: 5 Easy Ways for Busy People to Develop Sustainable Habits Around Food, Exercise and Self-Care."* The book is available on Amazon. Go to http://viewbook.at/livehealthy.

- *"Get Fit and Healthy in Your Own Home in 20 Minutes or Less: An Essential Daily Exercise Plan and Simple Meal Ideas to Lose Weight and Get the Body You Want."* The book is available on Amazon. Go to http://viewbook.at/get-fit.

- *"Get Fit and Healthy on a Tight Schedule 2 Books in 1." The book is available on Amazon. Go to http://viewbook.at/get-fit2books.*

- *"Beat Your Menopause Weight Gain: Balance Hormones, Stop Middle-Age Spread, Boost Your Health and Vitality."* The book is available on Amazon. Go to http://viewbook.at/beat-menopause.

- *"Break the Binge Eating Cycle: Stop Self-Sabotage and Improve Your Relationship With Food."* The book is available on Amazon. Go to http://viewbook.at/breakthebinge.

- *"Relaxation and Stress Management Made Simple: 7 Proven Strategies to Calm Your Mind, Stop Negative Thinking and Improve Your Life."* The book is available on Amazon. Go to http://viewbook.at/stressfree.

**Free Mini-Courses:**

- *Discover 10 Secrets of Successful Weight Loss*

- *This is How to Start Eating Less Sugar*

- *Learn How to Boost Your Energy – 11 Easy Ways*

- *Your Guide to a Happy and Healthy Menopause*

- *This is How to Lose Weight in Your 40's and Beyond*

***Free Courses Available at:***

www.silvanahealthandnutrition.com/course/